Accident and Emergency Radiology

Accident and Emergency Radiology
a survival guide

Nigel Raby MRCP, FRCR
Consultant Radiologist, Western Infirmary, Glasgow

Laurence Berman MRCP, FRCR
Consultant Radiologist, University Department of Radiology,
Addenbrookes Hospital and University of Cambridge, Cambridge

Gerald de Lacey, MA, FRCR
Consultant Radiologist, Northwick Park Hospital, London

Saunders
Edinburgh London New York Oxford Philadelphia
St Louis Sydney Toronto

Saunders
An imprint of Elsevier Science Limited

© 1995 W. B. Saunders Company Limited
© 1999 Harcourt Publishers Limited
© 2002 Elsevier Science Limited. All rights reserved.

Thirteenth printing 2003

This book is printed on acid-free paper

A catalogue record for this book is available from the British Library

ISBN 0-7020-1905-4

Line Drawings by Dr Laurence Berman using MacDraw Pro on Apple Macintosh
Typeset & Layout by Claire Gilman
Printed in the United Kingdom at the University Press, Cambridge

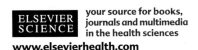

ELSEVIER SCIENCE your source for books,
journals and multimedia
in the health sciences
www.elsevierhealth.com

CONTENTS

FOREWORD

In an acute general hospital the Accident and Emergency Department is usually the busiest in terms of the numbers of patients seen. Staffing in the UK has improved dramatically over the last two decades and most departments are now led by a Consultant, – also most have Registrars or Senior Registrars. It is still the case, however, that the vast majority of patients seen in the Accident and Emergency Department are managed entirely by Senior House Officers who are relatively inexperienced. To add to the strain placed upon these young doctors is the fact that most conditions that will present to the minor side of the Accident Department will be completely new to them. The greatest difficulties faced by these doctors include deciding whether or not to x-ray the patient, and being confident in the interpretation of radiographs. Although there are many safety nets built into Accident and Emergency practice in the well-run departments designed so as to limit the problems caused by inaccurate interpretation of radiographs, mistakes will continue to occur given the large numbers of injured patients who attend on every day of the week.

It is with these thoughts in mind that I welcome the opportunity to write the Foreword for this excellent new book which I am sure will become rapidly popular, not only within Accident and Emergency Departments, but also amongst junior orthopaedic and radiology staff. It takes the young doctor through the basic principles of plain film radiography and explains the fundamentals of image formation, emphasizing and illustrating for instance the necessity of two views of an injury in any radiological examination associated with trauma. After this extremely clear introductory chapter the book moves on to describe the most appropriate radiographs for various injuries to the various parts of the body. This includes areas such as the chest where the reader will have had prior training, as well as, and much more importantly, those areas such as the face where almost no previous training will have been provided and which represent notoriously difficult regions for radiographic interpretation.

The approach to each chapter is logical. Each begins with the basic essential radiographs required to demonstrate a particular region followed by a review of the anatomy of the structure to be x-rayed. Then a description of the normal variants, which will in itself prevent many mis-diagnoses amongst junior doctors, followed by a series of examples, abnormalities, and in particular, fractures of various parts of the relevant region. The radiographs are well labelled so that there is no mistake in interpreting where the abnormality or abnormalities lie. Included in each chapter are descriptions and radiographs of common pitfalls in diagnosis, which will prepare the unwary and further help to avoid mistakes. Each chapter finishes with a series of key-points which will prove useful in reminding the reader of the most important features.

On appointment to their Senior House Officer post in Accident and Emergency, many junior doctors ask what books it might be useful to read before commencing. I have absolutely no doubt that as this book becomes increasingly popular, well-thumbed copies will appear in Accident and Emergency Departments up and down the country. When this occurs, the numbers of errors will be dramatically reduced, and in this way, patient care will equally dramatically improve.

David V. Skinner FRCS, Eng, FRCS, Ed, FRCS, Glas, FFAEM,
Consultant in Accident and Emergency Medicine
John Radcliffe Hospital
Oxford UK

16 September 1994

INTRODUCTION

This pocket guide has been written primarily for doctors with little or no experience in the Accident and Emergency Department and who are faced with problems of radiological interpretation at times when no other help or advice is readily available. There is ample evidence that inexperienced doctors do need this help: a recent survey (ref. 1) found that during night hours and at weekends 39% of clinically significant radiographic abnormalities were overlooked. This error rate is similar to that found in other studies.

Although designed primarily to assist doctors working in Accident and Emergency it is hoped that this guide will be of value to others in training, such as orthopaedic surgeons and radiologists. The emphasis is on the detection of those abnormalities that are commonly overlooked or misinterpreted, and the guide does not attempt to provide a comprehensive text on all aspects of orthopaedic radiology. For example, some important abnormalities that are rarely missed – such as Colles' fractures – have been deliberately excluded.

The approach may seem dogmatic with occasional statements in need of qualification. But we stress that this is a guide for doctors who have to make decisions at times when expert help and advice may not be immediately at hand. For this reason caveats and exceptions have been kept to a minimum.

We have described simple and systematic schemes for scrutinizing radiographs. In addition, whenever there is a standard projection on which most abnormalities will be demonstrated, it is this radiograph that has been emphasised. For example it is common practice for three facial radiographs to be obtained following trauma (lateral, frontal and occipito-mental views). In practice most abnormalities are demonstrated on the occipito-mental view – which is therefore the only one described in detail.

We have omitted several traditional and time-honoured classifications, for example the Le Fort classification of facial fractures, either because surveys have shown that they are not always clear-cut (ref. 2), or because they do not in themselves determine whether the patient requires referral to a specialist.

Throughout the text we have assumed two important principles. Firstly, that radiological investigations should never replace careful clinical examination but should always be correlated with the physical signs. Secondly, that guidelines essential for the appropriate practice of radiology need to be applied. Guidelines and protocols will vary from country to country and from department to department depending on the available facilities and the preferences of the local consultants. Therefore we have suggested specific protocols in only a few instances.

We have included a glossary to elucidate simple everyday radiological terms that in our teaching experience have been unfamiliar and confusing to junior accident and emergency doctors. In addition there are differences in terminology between The

United Kingdom and North America. We have also included some of the more common synonyms.

How soon will Accident and Emergency radiology be altered by the rapid changes now occurring in diagnostic imaging? For example magnetic resonance imaging can already replace some conventional Accident and Emergency radiographic examinations. Similarly, electronic transmission of images allows several sites to be covered by a single radiologist, thereby reducing errors in interpretation (ref. 3). However, in practice the widespread adoption of these advances will not occur for some years, and even then an understanding of conventional imaging together with the application of simple and systematic schemes for assessing conventional radiographs will remain fundamental to clinical practice in the Accident and Emergency department.

References

1. Vincent CA, Driscoll PA, Audley R, Grant DS Accuracy of detection of radiographic abnormalities by junior doctors. *Arch Emerg Med* 1988 **5:** 101–109.

2. Nakumura T, Gross CW Facial fractures. *Arch Otolaryngol* 1973, **97:** 288–290.

3. Franken EA, Berbaum KS, Smith WL, Chang P, Driscoll C, Bergus G Teleradiology for consultation between practitioners and radiologists. *Ann NY Acad Sci* 1992, **670:** 277–280.

Acknowledgements

The authors are greatly indebted to Claire Gilman of WB Saunders. Her skill, patience and hard work have been invaluable. Grateful thanks also to Dr Tina Beaconsfield for labelling the illustrations on pages 16–19.

GLOSSARY AND SYNONYMS

Synonyms are marked *aka*.

UK terms are marked [1], USA terms are marked [2].

Accessory ossicles   Normal small bones which are not always present in all individuals. Particularly common in the foot. An accessory ossicle may be confused with a fracture fragment. The usual distinguishing feature is that an accessory ossicle has well corticated margins.

Accessory ossification centre   Secondary centres of ossification which are normal variants but do not occur in all individuals. They may be mistaken for fracture fragments (e.g. in the patella).

Accident and Emergency Department[1]   *aka* Accident Department.[1] Emergency Room.[2]

Adynamic ileus[2]   *aka* Paralytic ileus.[1]

AP   Antero-posterior. Indicates the direction of the x-ray beam as it passes through the patient.

Atelectasis   *aka* Collapse (pulmonary).

Avulsion fracture   A bone fragment or apophysis pulled away from the parent bone. Usually occurs at the site of insertion of a tendon or ligament. Occurs as a result of excessive muscle contraction, an abnormal degree of forced movement at a joint, or chronic stress (e.g. ischial tuberosity).

Axial radiograph   The x-ray beam is directed along a plane parallel to the long axis of the body. For example, axial view of the shoulder and axial view of the calcaneum.

Bankart lesion   A fracture of the anterior glenoid labrum involving bone, cartilage, or both together. A potential complication of anterior dislocation of the glenohumeral joint.

Bennett's fracture   *aka* Bennett's fracture – dislocation. Fracture of the ventral aspect of the base of the first metacarpal. Usually associated with dislocation of the first carpo-metacarpal joint.

Bucket handle fracture   *aka* Corner fracture. A triangular fragment of bone detached from the margin of the metaphysis of a long bone in the unfused skeleton. When seen in an infant this type of fracture is suggestive of a non-accidental injury (NAI).

Button battery   *aka* Disc battery. Used, for example, in watches and electronic calculators.

Calcaneum   *aka* Calcaneus.

Capitellum   *aka* Capitulum.

Comminuted fracture   Splintering or fragmentation of a bone into three or more parts.

Decubitus   The patient is recumbent. In a radiographic context it denotes that the patient is lying on his or her side. The term also implies that a horizontal beam radiograph has been obtained. This technique is commonly used to demonstrate intra-abdominal air or fluid in the pleural space.

Diastasis   Separation at a joint, or separation at a site of fibro-cartilaginous union. For example, the ankle mortice, the sacroiliac joint, or a skull suture.

Dynamic ileus[2]   *aka* Mechanical obstruction.[1]

ENT surgery   Ear, nose and throat surgery.

Epidural   *aka* Extradural.

Epiphyseal fusion   *aka* Epiphyseal closure. The epiphysis has fully ossified and merged with the metaphysis of the long bone. The age at which ossification commences and fusion eventually occurs varies from bone to bone; there is a slight variation in the age at which fusion occurs between males and females.

Galeazzi fracture-dislocation   *aka* Galeazzi fracture. A fracture of the radius associated with dislocation of the distal ulna.

Gamekeeper's thumb   *aka* Skier's thumb. Rupture of the ulnar collateral ligament of the first metacarpo-phalangeal joint.

Garter strapping   *aka* Buddy strapping. A method of immobilizing some phalangeal fractures; the injured digit is strapped to an adjacent uninjured digit.

Greenstick fracture   There is a break of one cortex only. Usually accompanied by some angulation at the fracture site.

Growth plate   *aka* Cartilaginous growth plate, Epiphyseal plate, Physis. The layer of cartilage between the metaphysis and epiphysis of an unfused long bone.

Hemidiaphragm   *aka* Dome of the diaphragm. There is only one diaphragm. It has two domes.

Hill Sachs deformity   *aka* Hill Sach's lesion. A compression fracture of the postero-lateral margin of the humeral head. A potential complication of anterior dislocation of the gleno-humeral joint.

Horizontal beam radiograph   *aka* Cross table radiograph. Denotes the orientation of the x-ray beam relative to the floor. The beam is parallel to the floor. This technique may be used to demonstrate a fluid level (e.g. knee, skull), or when a patient should not be moved from the supine position (e.g. lateral cervical spine radiograph following trauma).

Intestinal obstruction *aka* Ileus

Intravenous urogram (IVU) *aka* Excretory urogram, Intravenous pyelogram (IVP).

Irritable hip *aka* Transient synovitis, Toxic synovitis.

Isotope investigation *aka* Nuclear medicine investigation, Radionuclide scan, Scintiscan, Scintigraphy.

Javelin thrower's elbow Avulsion injury occurring in relation to the lateral (external) epicondyle of the humerus.

Junior Doctor[1] *aka* Resident.[2]

Lipohaemarthrosis Liquid fat and blood within a joint. Only demonstrable on a horizontal beam radiograph. Most commonly seen at the knee joint when marrow fat enters the joint via an intra-articular fracture and forms a fat-fluid level.

Little leaguer's elbow[2] Avulsion injury occurring in relation to the medial (internal) epicondyle of the humerus. Occurs most commonly in children – particularly in those involved in throwing sports, such as baseball pitching.

Lucent Denotes a dark line, or dark area, on a radiograph. Commonly used as a descriptive term when indicating that a fracture is identifiable by a lucent line (or lucency).

Lytic The opposite of sclerotic. Denotes an area on a bone radiograph which appears darker or blacker than the adjacent normal bone. Frequently used as a synonym for lucent.

March fracture *aka* Fatigue fracture, Stress fracture. The term March fracture is used in reference to a stress fracture of a metatarsal.

Mallet finger[1] *aka* Baseball finger.[2] A flexion deformity of a distal interphalangeal joint with or without a fracture at the base of the phalanx. The injury represents an avulsion of the extensor tendon.

Monteggia fracture–dislocation *aka* Monteggia fracture. A fracture of the ulna associated with dislocation of the head of the radius.

Non-accidental Injury (NAI) *aka* Battered baby syndrome, Battered child syndrome, Child abuse. Euphemism for a deliberate assault. Used in the context of an injury to a young child or infant.

Occipito-frontal radiograph (OF) *aka* Caldwell projection.

Occipito-mental radiograph (OM) *aka* Water's projection. A radiograph of the face obtained with the axis of the x-ray beam directed between the chin and the occiput. May be followed by a number (e.g. OM 30) which denotes the degree of angulation of the x-ray beam.

Odontoid peg *aka* The dens of the axis vertebra.

OPG *aka* Orthopantomogram, OPT, Panoramic view. A tomographic device specifically designed to demonstrate the mandible and part of the maxilla.

Osteochondral fracture The fracture fragment consists of a small piece of bone and cartilage. The cartilaginous component is invisible on the plain radiograph. For example, fracture of the dome of the talus.

PA Postero-anterior. Indicates the direction of the X-ray beam as it passes through the patient.

Paraspinal line *aka* Paravertebral stripe. An interface between the vertebrae and the adjacent lung seen on a frontal radiograph. Most commonly seen to the left side of the thoracic vertebral bodies. The line is composed of the visceral and parietal pleura as they wrap around the side of the vertebrae. Any process that displaces the pleura away from a vertebra may cause localized widening of the paraspinal line. Displacement in the context of trauma is usually due to a haematoma from a vertebral fracture.

Periosteal new bone formation *aka* Periosteal reaction, Subperiosteal new bone formation. The appearance of a thin white line along part of the shaft of a long bone which appears to be separated from the cortex by a small space. The periosteum is invisible on a radiograph, and the reaction (or new bone) is a layer of ossification deep to the invisible periosteum. The small space between the white line and the bone is due to elevation of the periosteum by blood, pus, or tumour. In the context of trauma a periosteal reaction implies that healing is occurring.

Plastic bowing fracture *aka* Bowing fracture. A type of long bone fracture which occurs in children. A series of microfractures causes the bone to bend with no obvious abnormality of the cortex. Occurs most commonly in the forearm bones.

Pulled elbow[1] *aka* Nursemaid's elbow.[2]

Radiographer[1] *aka* Radiographic technician.[2]

Renal colic *aka* Ureteral colic, Ureteric colic.

Salter–Harris fracture *aka* Epiphyseal fracture. The Salter-Harris classification: a description of the fractures which involve the epiphyseal plate – with particular reference to prognosis.

Scaphoid bone[1] *aka* Carpal navicular.[2]

Sclerotic Denotes a dense (white) line or area on a radiograph. This may be at the periphery or cortex of a bone (e.g. the sclerotic appearance of maturing callus surrounding a healing fracture), or traversing the shaft of a bone (e.g. an impacted fracture).

Skyline view A tangential radiograph of the knee which provides a supero-inferior view of the patella and patello-femoral joint.

Snuff box   *aka* Anatomical snuff box. The area on the radial side of the carpus formed where the extensor tendons of the thumb pass over the base of the first metacarpal. Tenderness at this site is frequently associated with a scaphoid fracture.

Spinal canal   *aka* Vertebral canal. The space surrounded by the bony ring formed by the vertebral body anteriorly, the pedicles laterally and the laminae postero-laterally.

Stress fracture   *aka* Fatigue fracture. A fracture resulting from minor but repeated injury.

Sudeck's atrophy   *aka* Reflex sympathetic dystrophy syndrome. Severe localized osteopenia most commonly occurring as a result of trauma with or without a fracture.

Suture   The junction between adjacent membranous bones which is separated by a narrow layer of fibrous tissue.

Suture diastasis   *aka* Spread suture. Abnormal widening or separation of a suture.

Swimmer's view   A lateral radiographic projection which is occasionally used to show the junction between the seventh cervical and first thoracic vertebrae. The name derives from the patient's position: one arm is fully extended whilst the other remains by the side. The position simulates that of a swimmer doing the back stroke or crawl.

Symphysis   A joint between adjacent bones lined by hyaline cartilage and stabilized by fibrocartilage and ligaments.

Synchrondrosis   The site of a persistent plate of cartilage between adjacent bones, at which little or no movement occurs.

Torus   A term used to describe a particular shape of architectural moulding. Used also to describe a type of long bone fracture seen in children.

Towne's view   Skull radiograph obtained with the x-ray beam angled so as to obtain a view of the occipital bone clear of the overlying facial bones.

Trapezium bone[1]   *aka* Greater multangular.[2]

Trapezoid bone[1]   *aka* Lesser multangular.[2]

Vertical beam radiograph   Denotes the orientation of the x-ray beam with respect to the floor. The beam is at right angles to the floor.

Well corticated   A term used to describe the appearance of the periphery of a bone (e.g. an accessory ossicle) where it is seen to have a dense smooth margin. This appearance contrasts with the incompletely corticated margin of a fracture fragment.

1 BASIC PRINCIPLES

THE RADIOGRAPHIC IMAGE

■ Photographic film exposed to x-rays appears dark; those areas not exposed to x-rays appear white or pale.

■ Tissues that lie in the path of the x-ray beam absorb (or block) x-rays to differing degrees, and these differences affect the appearance of the radiograph:

  ▨ *Bone* blocks most of the beam and appears *white*.

  ▨ *Soft tissue* partially blocks the beam and appears *grey*.

  ▨ *Fat* blocks even less of the beam and appears *a darker shade of grey*.

  ▨ *Air*-containing tissues (such as lung) block very little of the beam and so produce the *blackest* image of all.

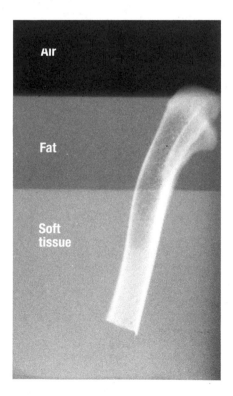

Figure 1.1. *Different tissues absorb the x-ray beam differently. Radiograph of a chicken leg (bone) partially submerged in a layer of vegetable oil (fat) floating on water (soft tissue). Note the difference in the blackening of the x-ray film.*

FRACTURES

■ A fracture may appear *as a lucent (black) line,* or as a *dense (white) line* on the x-ray film (Fig. 1.2).

■ When a fracture results in separation of bone fragments, the x-ray beam that passes through the gap is not absorbed by bone. This results in a dark (lucent) line on the film. On the other hand, bone fragments may overlap or impact into each other. The resultant increased thickness of bone absorbs more of the x-ray beam and so results in a whiter (sclerotic or more dense) area on the film.

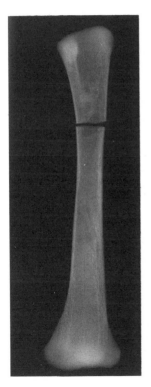
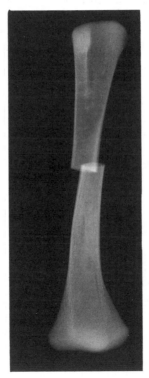
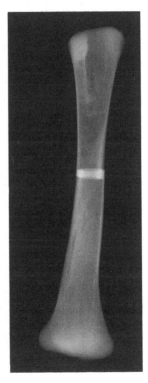

Figure 1.2. *Three fractures. On the left the fragments are distracted and the fracture is identified by a dark black line on the radiograph. In the centre and on the right the fragments overlap and the fracture is identified by a dense white line on the radiograph.*

THE PRINCIPLE OF TWO VIEWS

'One view only is one view too few'

■ Many fractures and some dislocations are not detectable on a single view (Fig. 1.3). Consequently, it is normal practice to obtain a minimum of two standard views, usually at right angles to each other.

■ Radiographic demonstration of a fracture requires that there is either some separation or impaction of the fragments. This requirement will not always be met and so it is inevitable that some fractures will not be shown on the two standard views (Fig. 1.4). The principle of two views is in effect a compromise, albeit a practical one.

■ Occasionally, at sites where fractures are known to be exceptionally difficult to detect (for example the scaphoid), it is routine practice to obtain more than two views.

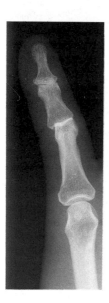 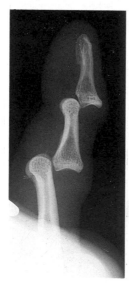

Figure 1.3. 'One view only is one view too few'. *Injured finger. The true extent of the injury is only evident from the lateral film.*

(a)

(b)

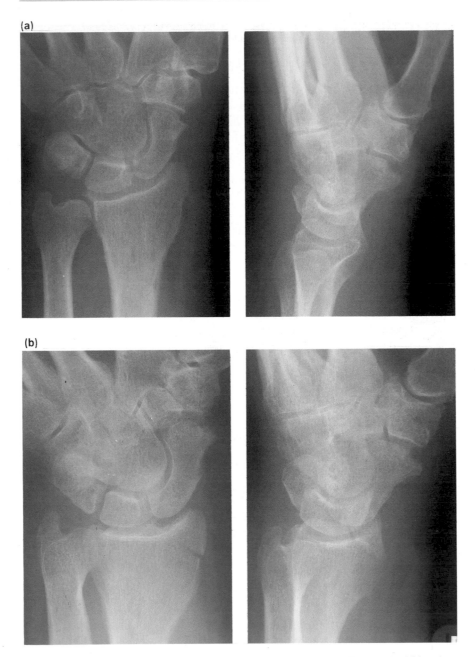

Figure 1.4. (a) *Fell on outstretched hand and injured the distal radius. The standard PA and lateral views appear within normal limits.* (b) *Same patient five minutes later. Two additional, slightly oblique, views. The fracture of the radius is now obvious. The practice of obtaining two views is itself a compromise; it is inevitable that the standard views will sometimes fail to show a fracture.*

PATIENT POSITION AND DIRECTION OF X-RAY BEAM

Sometimes the presence of a fluid level is the only clue to an important injury.

But:

■ A fluid level will only be shown when the radiograph is obtained using a horizontal x-ray beam (i.e. the beam is parallel to the floor). A vertical beam radiograph (i.e. the x-ray beam is at right angles to the floor) will not reveal a fluid level (Fig. 1.5).

■ The actual appearance of a fluid level will vary with the position of the patient.

■ Knowledge of the patient's position during radiography is important (Fig. 1.6) since the film may be obtained with the patient either supine or erect.

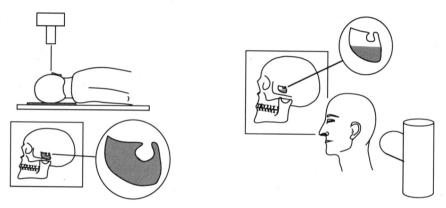

Figure 1.5. *Blood in the sphenoid sinus. A fluid level can only be demonstrated when a horizontal x-ray beam is used.*

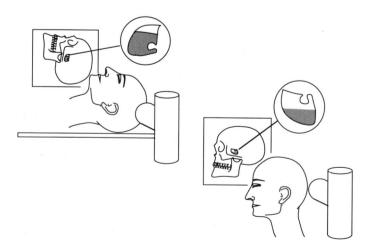

Figure 1.6. *Blood in the sphenoid sinus. Radiographs obtained with a horizontal beam. The orientation of a fluid level depends on the position of the patient.*

SOME NORMAL APPEARANCES CAN BE CONFUSING

Clinical correlation

The most important method of deciding whether a particular radiographic finding is significant is to correlate the appearance with the clinical examination. Indeed, it will often be necessary to re-examine the patient to look for swelling or tenderness at a particular site to weigh up the relevance of a particular radiographic appearance.

Vascular markings

A nutrient vessel may result in a dark (lucent) line in the cortex of a long bone (Fig. 1.7). This line may mimic a fracture. Typically, when seen in profile the line runs obliquely through one cortex only, from the inner to the outer margin. When seen *en face* at least one of the margins will appear sclerotic (dense).

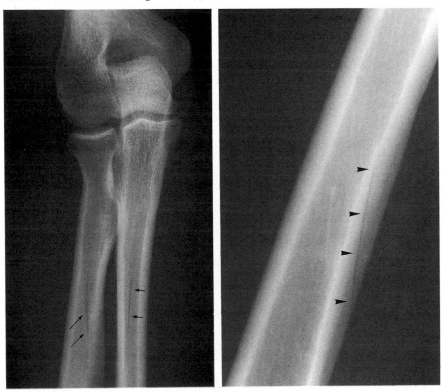

Figure 1.7. *Nutrient grooves in long bones. When seen* en face *a groove (ulna, small arrows) may mimic a fracture, but will usually have one slightly sclerotic margin (radius, large arrows). When seen in profile (femur, arrowheads) a groove is characteristically oblique and only involves one cortex of the bone.*

Accessory ossicles

There are many small bones that may occasionally mimic a fracture fragment. They are particularly common around the feet and ankles.

■ An ossicle has a well defined sclerotic (white) margin (Fig. 1.8). The bones adjacent to the ossicle are normal

■ a recent fracture fragment has at least one edge where the well defined sclerotic margin is absent (Fig. 1.9) or irregular. One of the adjacent bones will often show a similar irregular margin, representing the site from which the fragment has been detached.

Epiphyses and growth plates

■ Sometimes an epiphyseal line may be mistaken for a fracture. Distinguishing between normal and abnormal can be difficult (Fig. 1.10). When there is uncertainty it is best to seek expert advice. *Keats' Atlas* (ref. 1) will often be helpful.

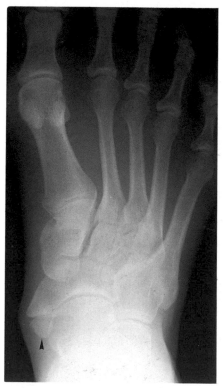

Figure 1.8. *Normal accessory ossicles need to be distinguished from fracture fragments. This accessory ossicle has a well-defined margin and the adjacent bones are normal.*

Figure 1.9. *The bone fragment (arrowhead) has a similar appearance to the accessory ossicle in Fig. 1.8, but the cortex is irregular and poorly defined. The adjacent bone is also abnormal. This is a fracture of the navicular.*

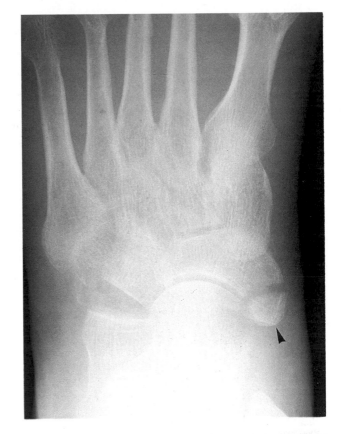

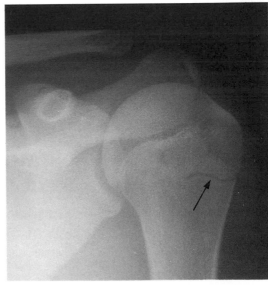

Figure 1.10. *Normal epiphyseal line in a 15-year-old boy.*

KNOWLEDGE OF NORMAL ANATOMY

The accurate interpretation of most x-ray images in the Accident Department depends in large part on a sound understanding of basic skeletal anatomy.

To test your knowledge, cover the captions and name the numbered bones and/or structures on the following radiographs.

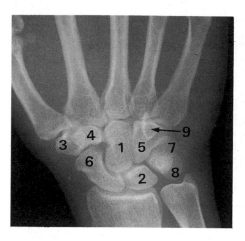

Figure 1.11. *PA view of the wrist. 1 = capitate, 2 = lunate, 3 = trapezium, 4 = trapezoid, 5 = hamate, 6 = scaphoid, 7 = triquetral, 8 = pisiform, 9 = hook of the hamate.*

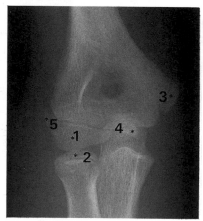

Figure 1.12. *AP view of a paediatric elbow. All are epiphyses: 1 = capitellum, 2 = head of radius, 3 = medial (or internal) epicondyle, 4 = trochlear, 5 = lateral (or external) epicondyle.*

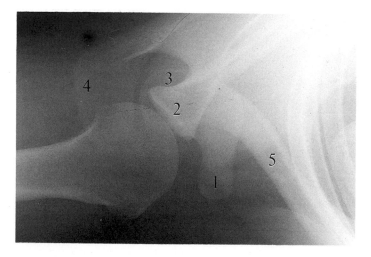

Figure 1.13. *Axial view of the shoulder. 1 = coracoid process of the scapula, 2 = glenoid, 3 = lateral end of the clavicle, 4 = acromion process of the scapula, 5 = clavicle.*

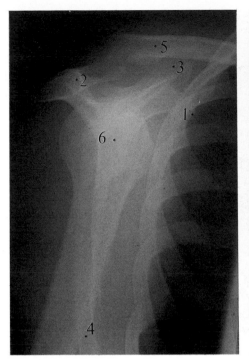

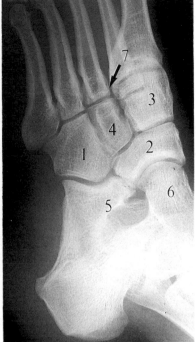

Figure 1.14. *The 'Y' view of a shoulder.*
1 = coracoid process of the scapula,
2 = acromion, 3 = superior margin of the
blade of the scapula, 4 = lateral margin of the
blade of the scapula, 5 = clavicle, 6 = head
of the humerus projected over the centre of
the glenoid.

Figure 1.15. *Oblique view of the foot.*
1 = cuboid, 2 = navicular, 3 = medial and
intermediate cuneiforms superimposed
over each other, 4 = lateral cuneiform,
5= calcaneum, 6 = talus, 7 = medial
margin of the base of the third metatarsal.

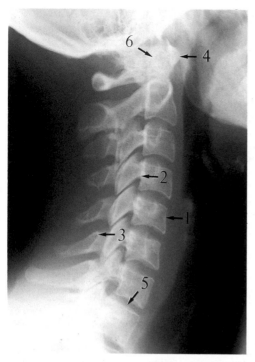

Figure 1.16. *Lateral view of the cervical spine. 1 = anterior margin of C5, 2 = pedicle of C4, 3 = base of the spinous process of C6 (or posterior margin of the spinal canal), 4 = anterior arch of C1, 5 = superior vertebral end plate of T1, 6 = odontoid peg.*

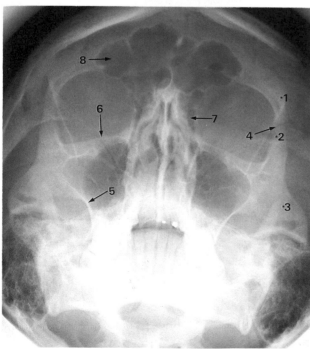

Figure 1.17. *OM view of the face. 1 = zygomatic process of the frontal bone, 2 = frontal process of the zygomatic bone, 3 = zygoma, 4 = synchondrosis (suture) between 1 and 2, 5 = lateral wall of the maxillary antrum, 6 = inferior wall of the orbit, 7 = ethmoid sinus, 8 = frontal sinus.*

Figure 1.18. *Skull. Towne's view. 1 = frontal and occipital bones superimposed on each other, 2 = margin of the foramen magnum.*

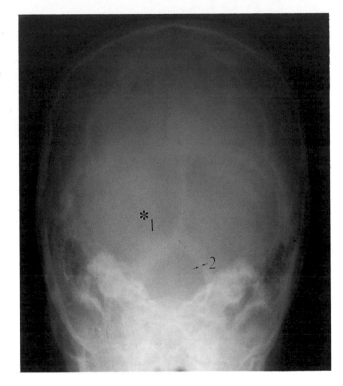

Reference

1. Keats TE. *Atlas of Normal Roentgen Variants That May Simulate Disease*, 5th edition. Year Book Medical Publishers, Chicago, 1991.

2 SKULL

Although inexperienced doctors are frequently anxious when evaluating skull films, abnormalities are not difficult to detect. There are only five things to look for, of which two are very rare. Most difficulties arise because some normal appearances can be mistaken for abnormalities.

BASIC RADIOGRAPHS

■ A lateral (Figs 2.1 and 2.2). Obtained with a horizontal x-ray beam.

■ Some centres obtain just one additional view. The particular projection will depend on the site of injury. If the injury is to the occipital bone then a Towne's view (Figs 2.3 and 2.4) is obtained. For injuries elsewhere an AP frontal view (Fig. 2.5) is taken.

■ In other centres it is routine practice to obtain two additional views irrespective of the site of injury: a frontal radiograph and a Towne's view.

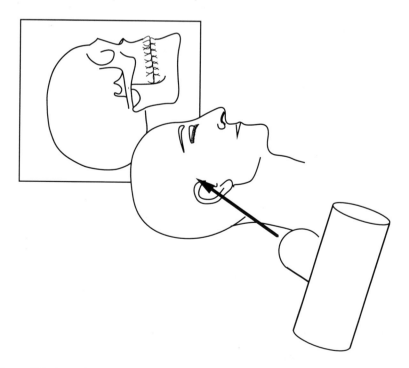

Figure 2.1. Lateral view. The patient is lying down. The importance of patient position and the use of a horizontal x-ray beam is described in Chapter 1 (page 12).

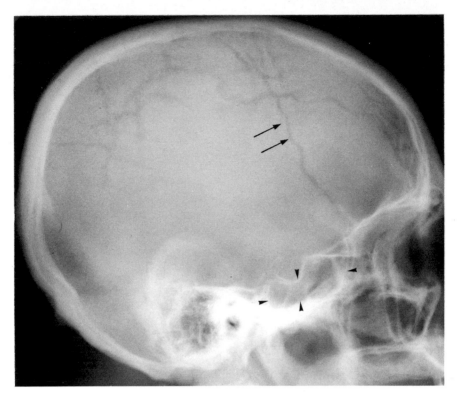

Figure 2.2. *Normal lateral view. Note: prominent vascular markings (arrows); position and appearance of the sphenoid sinus (arrowheads).*

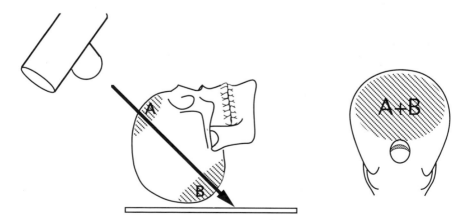

Figure 2.3. *Towne's view . This radiograph is obtained primarily to show the occipital bone. Note: the frontal and occipital bones are superimposed. Consequently a fracture through the frontal bone may also be seen on this view.*

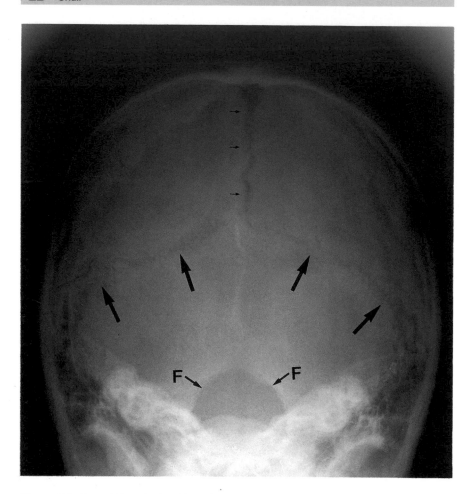

Figure 2.4. *Normal Towne's view. Note: the sagittal suture (small arrows); the lambdoid sutures are just visible (large arrows); the margin of the foramen magnum (F).*

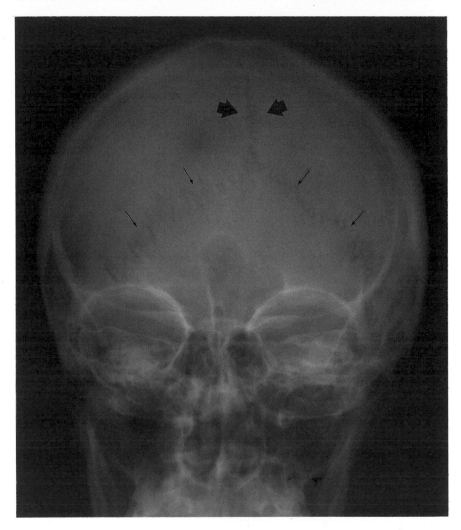

Figure 2.5. *Normal AP frontal radiograph. Note the sagittal suture (thick arrowheads); the lambdoid sutures (arrows).*

IMPORTANT ANATOMY

Be familiar with:

■ **The sutures**

▦ The position and appearance of the lambdoid, coronal and sagittal sutures (Figs 2.2, 2.4 and 2.5).

▦ The site of the common additional sutures. These occur most frequently in infants and children (Figs 2.6–2.8). Occasionally they persist in adults (Fig. 2.9).

▦ Accessory sutures. These are common, particularly in children. They may be unilateral, and thus incorrectly diagnosed as fractures. *Keats' Atlas of normal variants* (ref. 1) can often help in making the distinction.

■ **Vascular impressions**

▦ The sites of the common vessel markings (Fig. 2.2).

▦ The radiographic features which may assist in differentiating fractures from vascular markings (Table 2.1).

■ **The normal sphenoid sinus** (Fig. 2.10)

▦ In young children – it is not pneumatized.

▦ In adults – the appearance may vary.

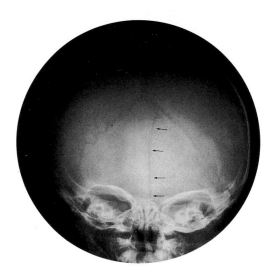

Figure 2.6. *Child. The metopic suture.*

Figure 2.7. *Child. Normal accessory suture. The intraparietal suture in this patient is unilateral. It can be bilateral.*

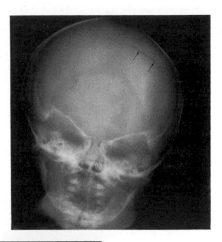

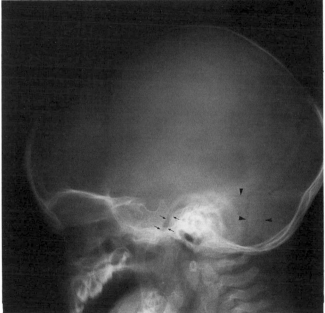

Figure 2.8. *Child. Normal synchondrosis between the sphenoid and occiput (arrows). Normal accessory sutures (arrowheads) should not be misinterpreted as fractures.*

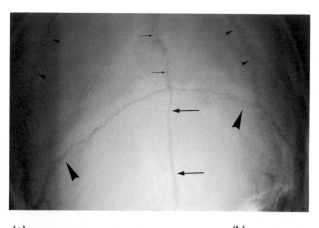

Figure 2.9. *Slightly rotated Towne's view showing an additional suture (large arrows). This is the metopic suture in the frontal bone which has persisted into adult life. Other normal sutures are also shown: sagittal suture (small arrows), lambdoid suture (small arrowhead), and coronal suture (large arrowhead).*

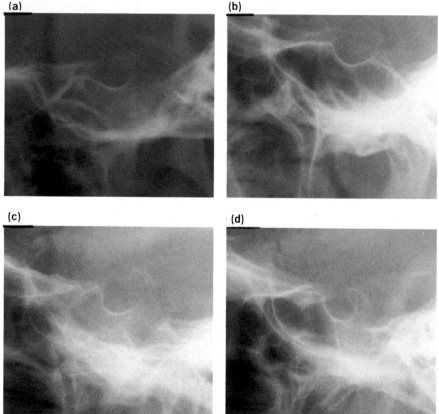

Figure 2.10. *Variable appearance of normal sphenoid sinus. Variation occurs because of age and also because of individual differences in pneumatization.* **(a)** *is a child and the sphenoid sinus has not yet begun to pneumatize;* **(b)** *is an adult and the sinus is well pneumatized;* **(c)** *is an adult but shows virtually no pneumatization;* **(d)** *is partly pneumatized and has resulted in an appearance which may be mistaken for a fluid level .*

Table 2.1. It is often very difficult to distinguish fractures from vascular markings. The following differences may help.

Fracture	Vascular marking
▣ Frequently appear black, because both inner and outer tables are involved.	▣ Appear grey, because only the inner table is thinned (Fig. 2.11).
▣ Branches do not taper uniformly.	▣ Branches *decrease* in size peripherally.
▣ Absence of a well defined white (sclerotic) margin.	▣ Sclerotic margins.

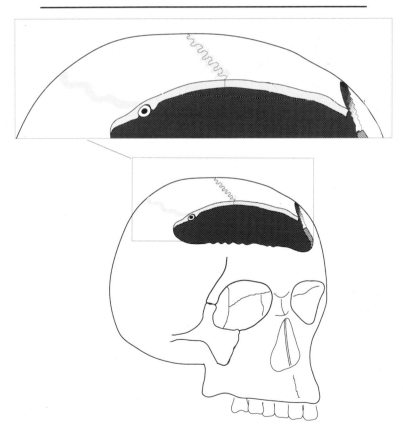

Figure 2.11. *A blood vessel (left) grooves the inner table of the skull only. The resultant marking appears as a grey line on the radiograph. A fracture (right) involves the full thickness of the skull. This often results in a very black line on the radiograph.*

INJURIES

Inspect the radiographs systematically:

Step 1

Scrutinize that part of the radiograph which corresponds to the site of injury, using a bright light if necessary.

Step 2

Examine the radiographs for three important abnormalities:

■ *A linear fracture* (Figs 2.12 and 2.13).

■ *A depressed fracture.* This appears as a dense (white) area due to overlapping bone fragments (Figs 2.14 and 2.15).

■ *A fluid level in the sphenoid sinus.* This is only detectable on a lateral film which has been taken with a horizontal beam.

   ▪ A fluid level indicates that a basal skull fracture is present (Figs 2.16–2.18). This may be the only abnormality on the radiograph. Detection of a fluid level will affect management since a fracture involving the sphenoid sinus is a compound fracture.

Step 3

Look for two exceptionally rare abnormalities:

■ **Intracranial air.** This is seen as an unusual lucency in the basal cisterns, in the cerebral sulci, or in the lateral ventricles (Fig. 2.19). The air usually results from a fracture involving a sinus; occasionally it may result from a penetrating injury.

■ **Lateral displacement of a calcified pineal.** The pineal gland should be no more than 3 mm to one side of the mid-line on the frontal or Towne's radiograph. Displacement of a calcified pineal is an exceptionally rare finding in a patient who attends with a seemingly mild head injury. Displacement indicates that a large intracranial haematoma is present.

Note: Difficulties for the inexperienced doctor most commonly arise when a normal appearance is mistaken for an abnormality. In practice a mistake along these lines will simply lead to a false positive diagnosis, which rarely has an adverse effect on patient management.

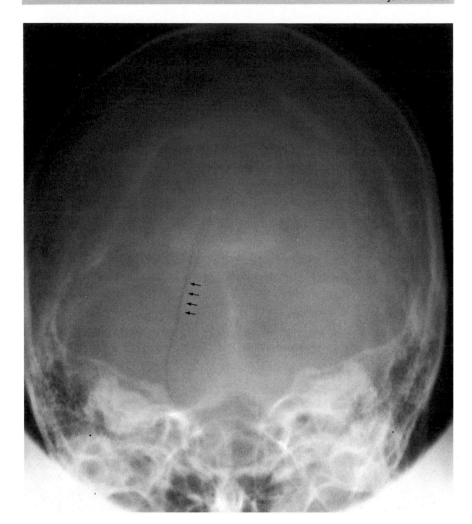

Figure 2.12. *Towne's view. A linear fracture through the occipital bone.*

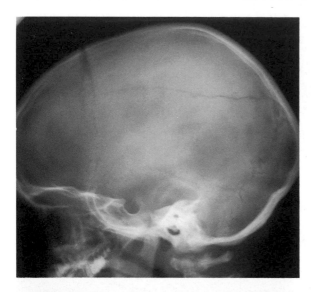

Figure 2.13. *Linear fracture through the parietal bone.*

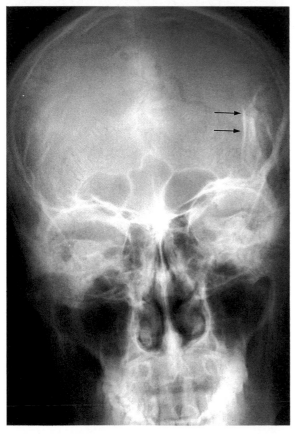

Figure 2.14. *A depressed fracture seen only as an area of dense bone.*

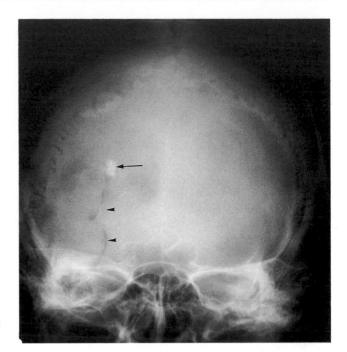

Figure 2.15. *A fracture with both linear (arrowheads) and depressed (arrow) components.*

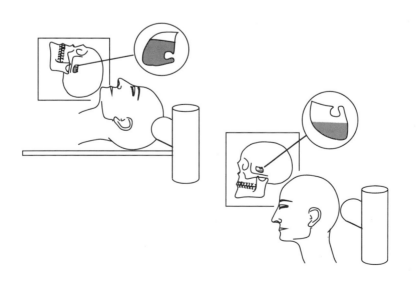

Figure 2.16. *The appearance of a fluid level in the sphenoid sinus will depend on the position of the patient (see page 12). It is important to know how the lateral view has been obtained.*

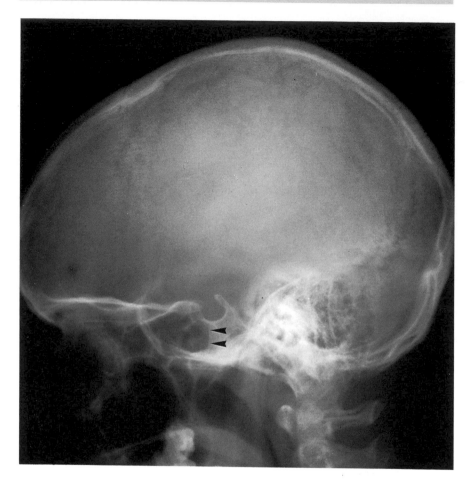

Figure 2.17. *Fluid level in the sphenoid sinus. This indicates a fracture through the base of the skull. Radiograph obtained with the patient supine and using a horizontal x-ray beam.*

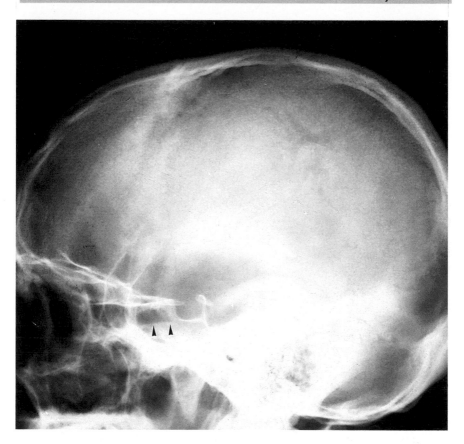

Figure 2.18. *Fluid level in the sphenoid sinus is the only radiographic evidence of a basal skull fracture in this patient. Radiograph obtained with the patient sitting up.*

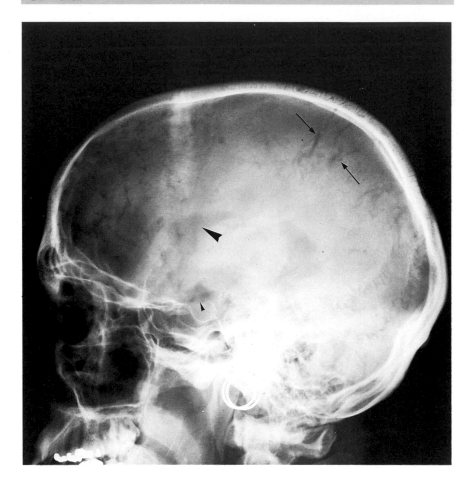

Figure 2.19. *Intracranial air resulting from a fracture which involved the sphenoid sinus. Air is present in the cerebral sulci (arrows), in a lateral ventricle (large arrowhead), and in the basal cisterns (small arrowhead).*

KEY POINTS

■ Lateral views are invariably taken with a horizontal x-ray beam.

■ Be familiar with the appearance of:

■ all the normal sutures;

■ normal vascular markings.

■ *Keats' Atlas* (ref. 1) can be very helpful in identifying the normal variants which may mimic fractures.

Look for:

■ **Three important abnormalities**

linear fracture – lucent (black on radiograph);

depressed fracture – dense (white on radiograph);

fluid level in the sphenoid sinus.

■ **Two *very rare* abnormalities**

intracranial air;

shift of a calcified pineal.

Reference

1. Keats TE. *Atlas of Normal Roentgen Variants That May Simulate Disease*, 5th edition. Year Book Medical Publishers, Chicago, 1991.

3 FACE

The face

The number of views will vary between hospitals. The following practice is common.

■ A tilted up frontal radiograph, known as an occipito-mental (OM) (Fig. 3.1).

■ An additional OM view with increased upward tilt of the face, known as an OM 30° (Fig 3.2).

■ A lateral.

Because of superimposition of bones the radiographic anatomy on the lateral view can be very difficult to evaluate. In practice, this view rarely adds any important information to the initial assessment of the patient.

Concentrate on the OM views.

The mandible

■ Many accident departments use a device which provides a tomographic unwrapped view of the entire mandible (Fig. 3.4). This is often referred to as an orthopantomogram (OPG). This will show virtually all mandibular fractures.

■ If OPG equipment is not available it is normal practice to obtain three plain films: a PA and two obliques. The PA view (Fig. 3.5) demonstrates the body of the mandible, and also provides tangential views of the mandibular rami including the necks of the condyles. The oblique views (Fig. 3.6) demonstrate the body and ramus of the mandible on each side.

The nasal bone

A routine request for radiography is not necessary even if a fracture is certain on clinical grounds (ref. 1). In general, radiography is only indicated when requested by a specialist surgeon.

IMPORTANT ANATOMY

The face

Interpretation of the OM views is straightforward, despite the apparently complicated anatomy. Note:

■ The orbital margins, frontal sinuses, zygomatic arches and maxillary antra are well demonstrated with minimal overlap from other bony structures (Figs 3.1 and 3.2).

■ The zygomatic arches, frequent sites of injury, are easy to identify. They may be likened to the trunks of two elephants, facing right and left (Fig. 3.3).

■ The OM projections provide a normal (uninjured) side for comparison.

Figure 3.1. *The OM view. This provides an excellent demonstration of the upper as well as the middle third of the face.*

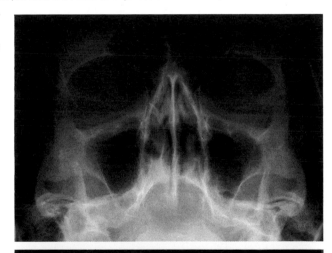

Figure 3.2. *The OM 30° view. The upper third of the face is not so well shown, but this is the best view for demonstrating the zygomatic arches and the walls of the maxillary antra.*

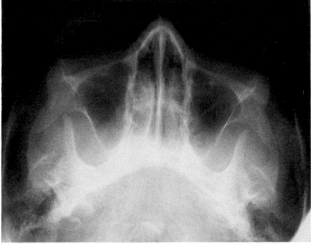

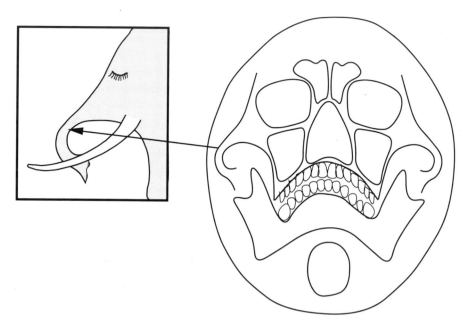

Figure 3.3. Each zygomatic arch can be likened to an elephant's trunk on the OM views.

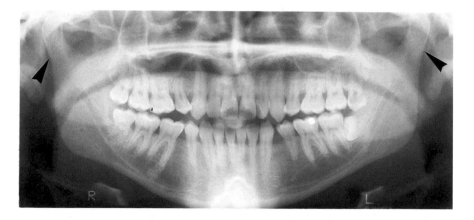

Figure 3.4. An OPG view to show the mandible. The mandibular condyles (arrowheads) are well demonstrated.

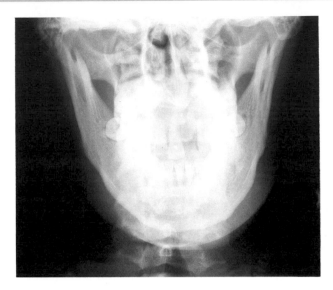

Figure 3.5. *PA mandible. The condyles are difficult to see because of superimposition of bones.*

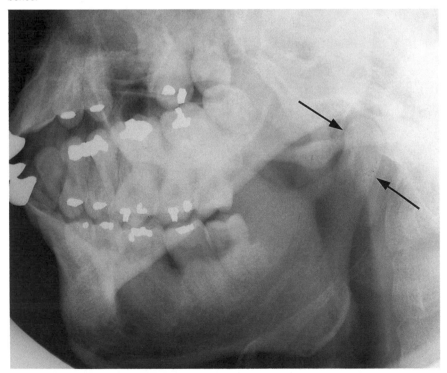

Figure 3.6. *An oblique view demonstrates the right ramus and condyle (arrows) of the mandible.*

A SYSTEM FOR INSPECTING THE OM VIEWS

McGrigor described how the OM films can be assessed by means of a series of lines traced over the radiograph (ref. 2). The following modified version of McGrigor's approach is recommended.

McGrigor's three lines

■ Trace three lines on the OM views (Fig. 3.7).

■ As the lines are drawn compare the injured with the uninjured side.

■ The soft tissues above and below these three lines should also be scrutinized. A fluid level or other soft tissue abnormality may be evidence of an underlying bone injury.

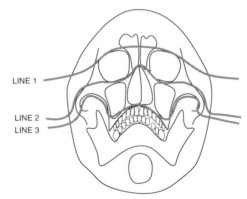

Figure 3.7. *McGrigor's three lines.*

Line 1

Start outside the face, tracing through the synchondrosis (i.e. the suture) between the frontal bone and zygomatic bone at the lateral margin of the orbit. Follow across the forehead, assessing the superior orbital margin and the frontal sinus. Continue on to the other side of the radiograph following the same landmarks (Fig. 3.8). The injured and uninjured sides should be compared.

Look for:

■ fractures;

■ widening of the zygomatico-frontal suture;

■ fluid level (haemorrhage) in a frontal sinus.

Pitfall: The width of the normal zygomatico-frontal suture is variable. Compare the injured with the uninjured side.

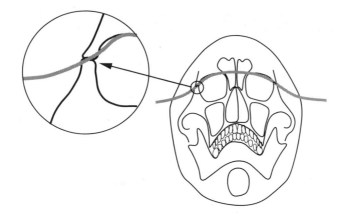

Figure 3.8. *McGrigor's line 1. Note the position of the normal zygomatico-frontal suture.*

Line 2

Starting outside the face, trace upwards along the superior border of the zygomatic arch (up the elephant's trunk), crossing the body of the zygoma, and continuing on to the inferior margin of the orbit. Follow the contour of the nose, and in a similar way on to the other side of the radiograph (Fig. 3.9).

Look for:

■ Fractures of the zygomatic arch (Fig. 3.10.)

■ A fracture through the inferior rim of the orbit.

■ A soft tissue shadow in the superior aspect of the maxillary antrum (see page 46: blow-out fracture).

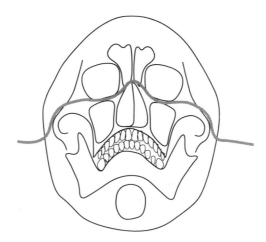

Figure 3.9. *McGrigor's Line 2.*

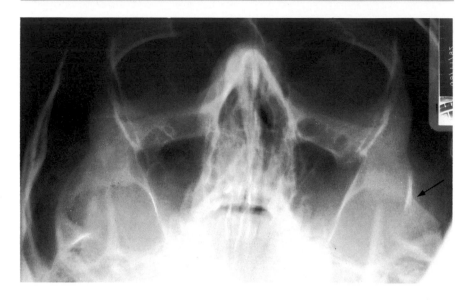

Figure 3.10. *Tracing McGrigor's line 2 reveals a step (fracture) in the normal curve of the left zygomatic arch (elephant's trunk). Compare this with the appearance of the uninjured right zygomatic arch.*

Line 3

Starting outside the face, trace along the inferior margin of the zygomatic arch (under the elephant's trunk), and down the lateral wall of the maxillary antrum. Continue along the inferior margin of the antrum, across the maxilla including the roots of the teeth (look very carefully – fractures of this part of the maxilla are extremely difficult to detect). Follow the same structures on to the other side of the face (Fig. 3.11).

Look for:

■ fractures of the zygoma and of the lateral aspect of the maxillary antrum (Fig. 3.12);

■ a fluid level in the maxillary antrum. In the context of trauma assume a fluid level to represent haemorrhage from a fracture (Fig. 3.13).

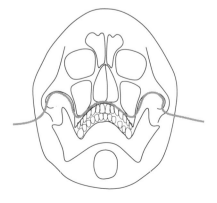

Figure 3.11. *McGrigor's line 3.*

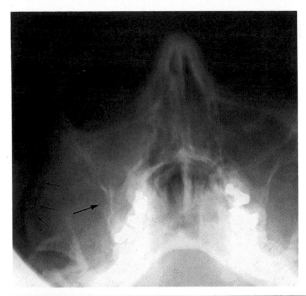

Figure 3.12. Tracing McGrigor's line 3 reveals fractures of the zygomatic arch (small arrows), and of the lateral wall of the maxillary antrum (large arrow).

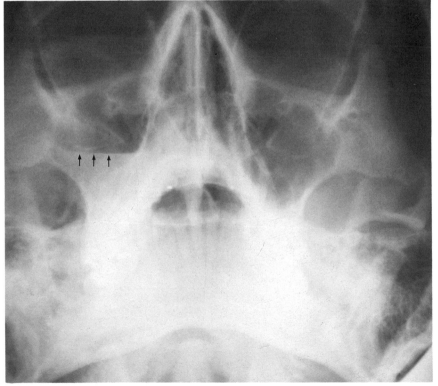

Figure 3.13. Fluid level in the maxillary antrum. Following trauma this is most likely to be blood from a fracture. A fracture is not visible on this radiograph.

Tripod fracture

■ An isolated fracture of the zygomatic arch *is common.*

■ Isolated fractures through the zygomatico-frontal suture or through the body of the zygoma *are rare.* Fractures usually occur as part of a combination injury known as a tripod fracture (Fig. 3.14). This comprises:

1 Widening of the zygomatico-frontal suture.

2 Fracture of the zygomatic arch.

3 Fracture through the body of the zygoma. This is seen on the radiograph as a fracture of the inferior margin of the orbit and of the lateral wall of the maxillary antrum (Fig. 3.15).

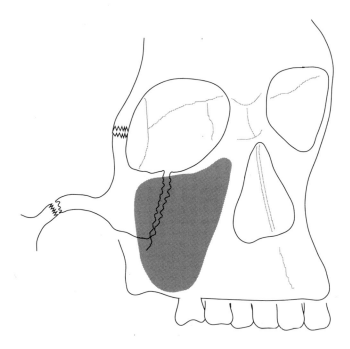

Figure 3.14. *Tripod fracture. The shaded area indicates the maxillary antrum. The fracture through the body of the zygoma will appear on the OM radiograph as fractures through the inferior wall of the orbit and through the lateral wall of the maxillary antrum.*

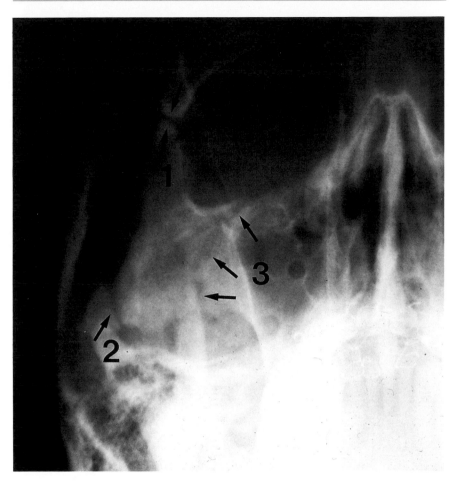

Figure 3.15. *Tripod fracture. There are fractures through the zygomatico-frontal suture (1), the zygomatic arch (2), and through the body of the zygoma (3).*

Blow-out fracture

■ Results from a direct compressive force (Fig. 3.16) to the globe (e.g. from a squash ball).

■ A fracture of the strong inferior orbital rim is not a feature of this injury.

    ▦ The walls of the orbit fracture at the weakest points. These are the thin plates of bone which form the floor of the orbit (i.e. the roof of the maxillary antrum), and the medial wall of the orbit (i.e. the lateral margin of the ethmoid sinus).

    ▦ Some of the orbital contents may herniate downwards through the orbital floor (Fig. 3.17). This has been likened to an opaque tear drop hanging from the roof of the antrum. This teardrop may be the only radiographic evidence of a blow out fracture and it will be detected when McGrigor's second line is traced (Fig. 3.18). The actual fracture fragments are often difficult to identify.

    ▦ Occasionally not even a teardrop can be identified. A fracture through the wall of the maxillary or ethmoid sinus may only be detected because air has entered the orbit. The air can sometimes be seen on the radiograph. This has given rise to the term 'the black eyebrow sign' (Fig. 3.19).

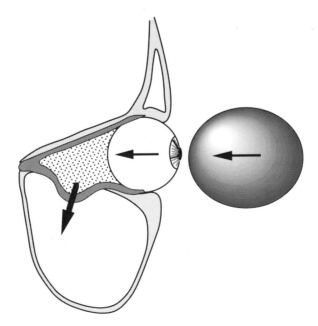

Figure 3.16. *Blow out fracture. Increased intraorbital pressure has caused a fracture of the thin plate of bone which forms the floor of the orbit. Fat and muscle has herniated downwards, resulting in an appearance rather like a tear drop in the roof of the maxillary antrum.*

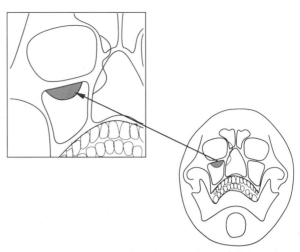

Figure 3.17. *Blow out fracture. The soft tissue tear-drop in the roof of the maxillary antrum represents herniated orbital contents (dark shading). Herniation through the medial wall of the orbit into the ethmoid sinus (light shading) commonly occurs but is hard to detect on the radiographs.*

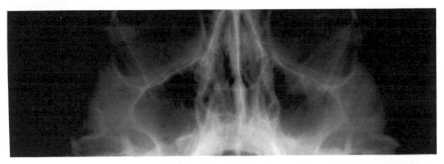

Figure 3.18. *Blow out fracture. Soft tissue (the tear-drop) is seen hanging from the roof of the maxillary antrum. The radiograph above is the OM view. The radiograph on the right is a tomogram.*

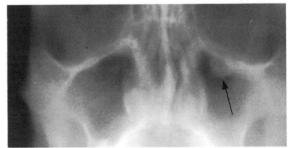

Figure 3.19. *Blow out fracture. The radiographic appearances are entirely within normal limits apart from the black eyebrow sign (arrows). This appearance is due to air from a sinus entering the orbit. CT examination later confirmed a fracture through the roof of the maxillary antrum.*

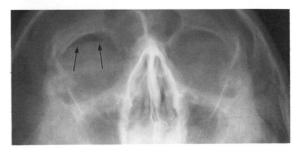

Mandibular fractures

■ Regard the mandible as a rigid bony ring. When a bony ring is broken it is very common for two fractures to occur (Fig. 3.20).

■ Examine the mandibular condyles carefully. Fractures are common but they may be very subtle. It is particularly important that the radiological inspection is correlated with the precise site of clinical injury.

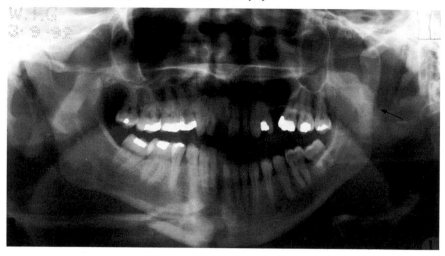

Figure 3.20. *Fracture through the body of the mandible. There is a second fracture (arrow) through the left condylar process. This condyle is also dislocated.*

KEY POINTS

■ **Concentrate on the OM views.**

▨ Be familiar with the 'elephant's trunk' appearance of the zygomatic arch.

▨ Trace the three McGrigor's lines looking for bony and soft tissue abnormalities.

▨ Compare the injured side with the normal side

▨ blow out fracture: look for soft tissue swelling in the roof of the maxillary antrum.

■ Regard the mandible as a bony ring. Solitary fractures are rare. Two fractures are common.

References

1. de Lacey GJ, Wignall BK, Hussain S, Reidy JR. The Radiology of nasal injuries: problems of interpretation and clinical relevance. *Brit J Radiol* 1977, **50:** 412–414.

2. McGrigor DB, Campbell W. The Radiology of war injuries. Part VI. Wounds of the face and jaw. *Brit J Radiol* 1950, **23:** 685–696.

4 SHOULDER

BASIC RADIOGRAPHS

- An AP view is standard in all hospitals (Fig. 4.1).

- The second view will vary. One of the following is common:

  - *Axial view.* This is equivalent to looking up into the patient's armpit (Fig 4.2). It does have some disadvantages:

    - ❏ abducting the injured arm may be painful for the patient;

    - ❏ pain may make it difficult to obtain a technically optimal radiograph.

  - *Y view.* A lateral scapular radiograph (Fig 4.3). Some centres prefer this projection to the axial view because it:

    - ❏ does not cause the patient any discomfort;

    - ❏ is technically easy to obtain;

    - ❏ is easy to interpret.

  - *Oblique axial view.* This view (refs 1, 2) does have advantages:

    - ❏ the patient's arm is not moved;

    - ❏ bone fragments detached from the glenoid are easy to detect;

    - ❏ it is easy to interpret (Fig 4.4).

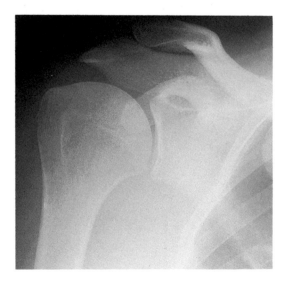

Figure 4.1. *The standard AP view.*

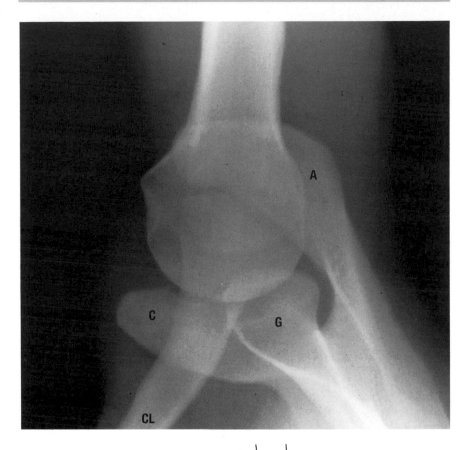

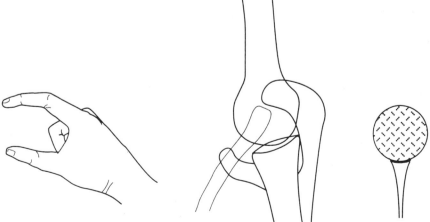

Figure 4.2. *The axial or armpit view. A, acromion; C, coracoid; G, glenoid; CL, clavicle. The head of the humerus sits on the glenoid like a golf ball on a tee. Orientation is easy: the 'fingers' (i.e. the acromion and coracoid processes) always point anteriorly.*

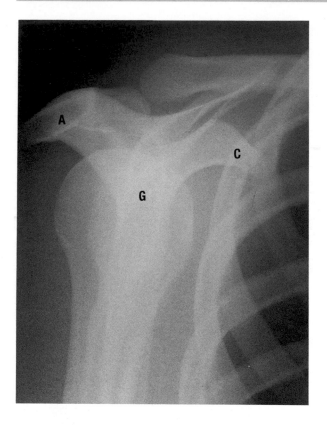

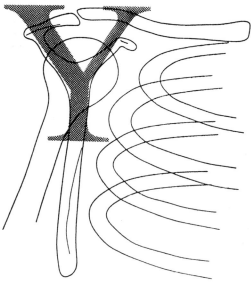

Figure 4.3. *The Y view. The humeral head overlies the centre of the glenoid (G). The Y is formed by the junction of the scapular blade, coracoid (C) and acromion (A).*

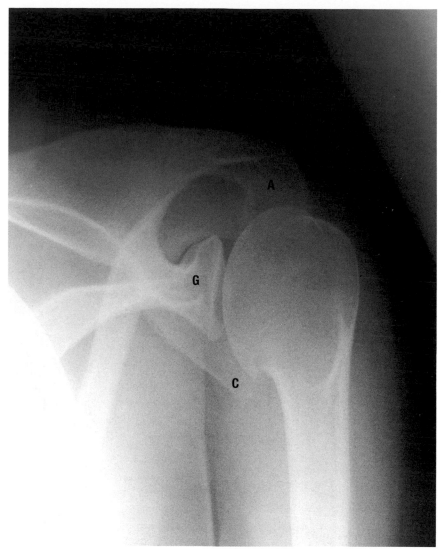

Figure 4.4. *The oblique axial view (A, acromion; C, coracoid; G, glenoid).*

IMPORTANT ANATOMY

AP view

■ The humeral head is not symmetrical. It has a configuration which is more like the head of a walking stick (Figs 4.1 and 4.5).

■ The articular surfaces of the humerus and the glenoid parallel each other (Figs 4.1 and 4.5).

■ The inferior aspects of the acromion and clavicle should be at the same level (Fig. 4.1).

Axial (armpit) view

■ The humerus sits on the glenoid like a golf ball on a tee (Fig 4.2).

■ The acromion and coracoid processes (these can be likened to 'fingers') point forwards/anteriorly.

Y view

■ **Anterior** is on the side of the rib cage.

■ **The stem of the Y** is the blade of the scapula.

■ **The limbs of the Y** are the coracoid and the acromion.

■ The junction of the stem and the limbs of the Y indicates the centre of the glenoid.

■ The head of the humerus should overlap the centre of the glenoid (Fig 4.3).

Oblique axial view

■ *Note*: the x-ray tube is positioned above the shoulder with the x-ray beam angled at 45 degrees to the vertical and this produces a rather bizarre view.

■ The superior aspect of the humerus and the glenoid fossa are well shown (Fig. 4.4). Small fractures at these sites are therefore easy to detect.

NORMAL VARIANTS

■ In the unfused skeleton the normal humeral growth plate frequently appears as two lucent lines (Fig. 4.6). These may be misinterpreted as fractures.

■ The tips of the acromion and coracoid ossify from separate centres. These do not always fuse. They may be mistaken for fractures, especially on the armpit view.

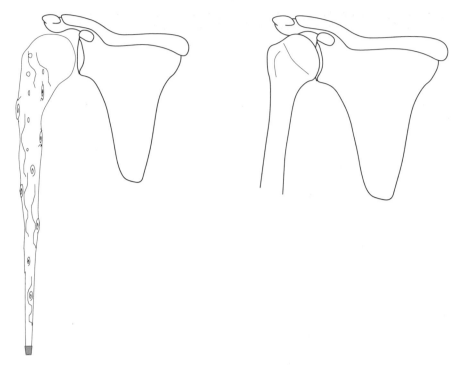

Figure 4.5. *On the AP view the normal humeral head has a configuration rather like that of a walking stick.*

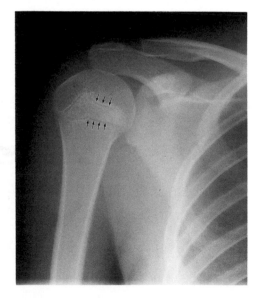

Figure 4.6. *Normal epiphyseal lines in a 14-year-old.*

INJURIES

Fractures

■ Fractures are common involving:

   ▨ The neck of the humerus and the greater tuberosity (Fig. 4.7).

   ▨ The head of the humerus and the glenoid rim as complications of an anterior dislocation (Figs 4.8 and 4.9).

   ▨ The clavicle (Fig. 4.10). This is one of the few bones which is not routinely radiographed in two projections. The majority of fractures involve the middle third.

■ A fracture through the body of the scapula is uncommon but is easy to overlook (Fig. 4.11).

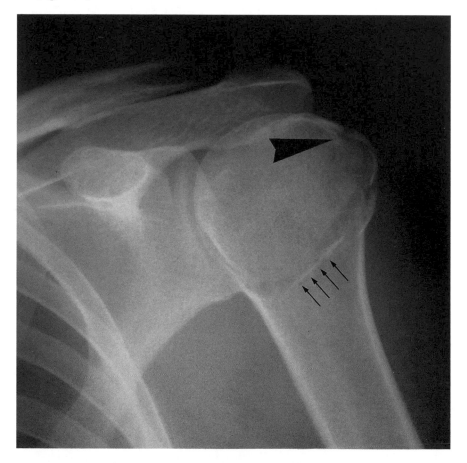

Figure 4.7. *Fractures of the humeral neck (small arrows), and greater tuberosity (arrow head).*

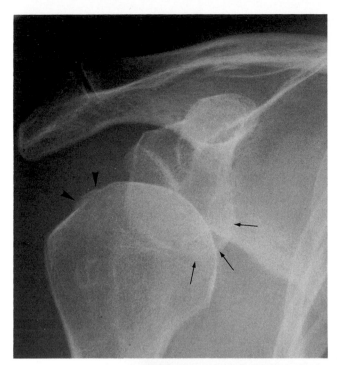

Figure 4.8. *Common complications of an anterior dislocation: fracture of the glenoid (arrows), and a fracture through the greater tuberosity (arrowheads).*

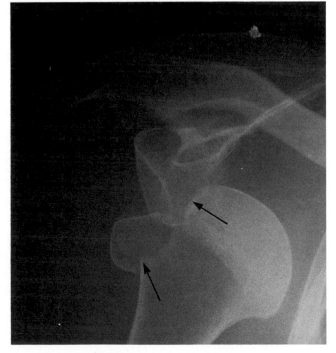

Figure 4.9. *A common complication of an anterior dislocation: fracture of the humeral head and neck.*

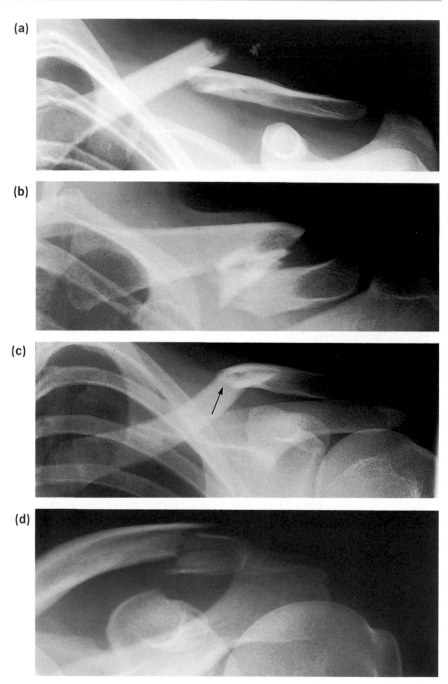

Figure 4.10. *Fractures of the clavicle. Most involve the middle third* **(a)***; some are comminuted* **(b)***; most are easy to detect* **(a, b)***; some are more difficult to detect* **(c)***; a few involve the outer third* **(d)***.*

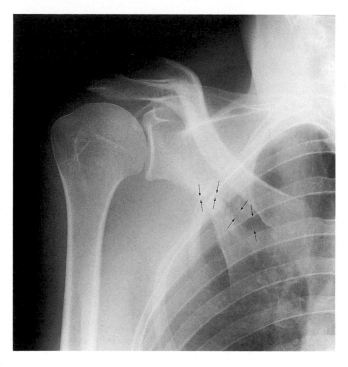

Figure 4.11. *Injured shoulder. Normal joint, but the fracture through the body of the scapula was overlooked.*

Anterior dislocation

■ Very common. Rarely overlooked.

■ The following appearances are characteristic (Figs 4.12–4.15):

  ▓ The head of the humerus lies under the coracoid process on the AP view.
  ▓ The armpit and the oblique axial views show the golf ball (head of the humerus) anterior to the tee (the glenoid).
  ▓ The Y view shows the head to be displaced anteriorly. It no longer covers the glenoid (the centre of the Y).

■ Following manipulation, a repeat film should always be obtained to confirm reduction.

■ Scrutinize all films, particularly the post-reduction film for fractures. Common complications (Figs 4.8 and 4.9) are fractures to:

  ▓ the anterior lip of the glenoid;
  ▓ the posterolateral aspect of the head of the humerus.

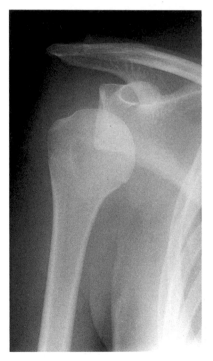

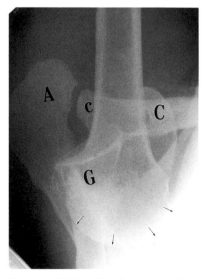

Figure 4.13. *Armpit radiograph. A = acromion, C = coracoid, c = clavicle, G = glenoid. The humeral head (the golf ball) is indicated by the arrows and lies anterior to the glenoid (the tee). The acromion and coracoid (the fingers) point anteriorly.*

Figure 4.12. *Anterior dislocation. Typical appearance on the AP radiograph. Note the subcoracoid position of the humeral head.*

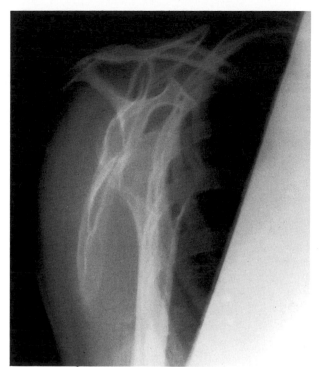

Figure 4.14. *Anterior dislocation. Y view. The humeral head lies anterior to the glenoid (the centre of the Y).*

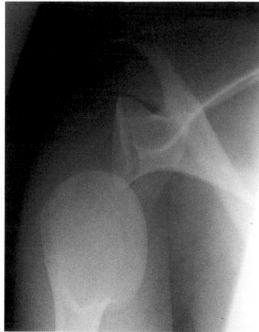

Figure 4.15. *Anterior dislocation. Oblique axial view. The humeral head lies anterior to the glenoid.*

Posterior dislocation

■ *Uncommon.* Less than 5% of shoulder dislocations. Frequently overlooked.

■ Often results from severe muscle spasm during an epileptic fit or from an electric shock.

■ The following appearances occur.

  ▪ *On the AP view* the head of the humerus may maintain a normal shape. In other instances the contour is more that of a light bulb (Fig. 4.16) than that of a walking stick. This change in contour is due to rotation.

  ▪ *On the armpit and axial oblique view* (Figs 4.17 and 4.18) the golf ball (head of the humerus) lies posterior to the tee (glenoid).

  ▪ *On the Y view* the head of the humerus lies posterior to the junction of the limbs of the Y (Fig. 4.19).

Pitfall: occasionally, a normal AP shoulder will show a light-bulb configuration (Fig. 4.20) and not that of a walking stick (Figs 4.1 and 4.5). This is because a normal but painful shoulder may be held in some degree of internal rotation (Fig. 4.21) and thus may mimic a posterior dislocation (Fig. 4.20). The appearance on the second view is crucial and will exclude a posterior dislocation.

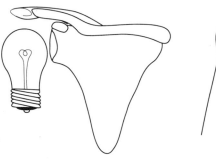
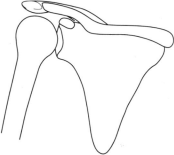

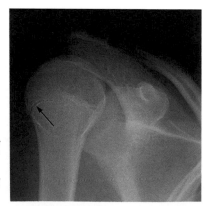

Figure 4.16. *Posterior dislocation. On the AP view the head of the humerus often adopts the shape of a lightbulb. It no longer resembles the head of a walking stick. (Note: the arrow indicates the normal epiphyseal line in an adolescent.)*

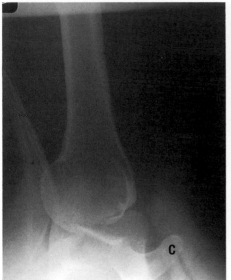
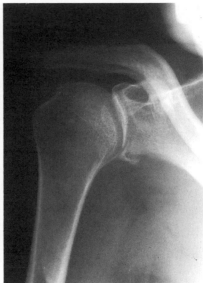

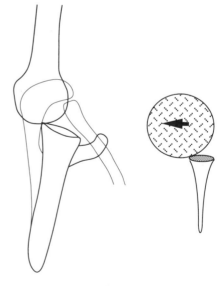

Figure 4.17. *Posterior dislocation. In this instance the humeral head resembles a walking stick on the AP view. On the armpit view the humeral head lies posterior to the glenoid – the golf ball is off the tee. C = coracoid.*

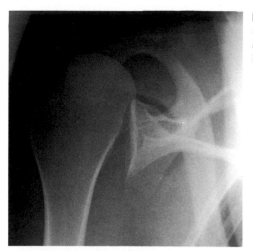

Figure 4.18. *Posterior dislocation. Oblique axial view. The head of the humerus lies posterior to the glenoid fossa.*

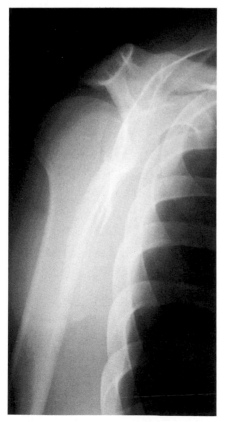

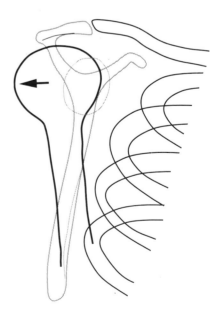

Figure 4.19. *Posterior dislocation. Y view. The humeral head lies behind the glenoid (the centre of the Y).*

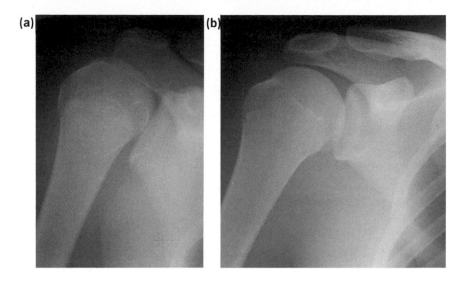

Figure 4.20. Pitfall: *In this instance the light-bulb appearance of the head of the humerus* **(a)** *is not due to a posterior dislocation. It is due to pain causing the humerus to be held in a position of internal rotation. A repeat film* **(b)** *shows the normal walking stick appearance.*

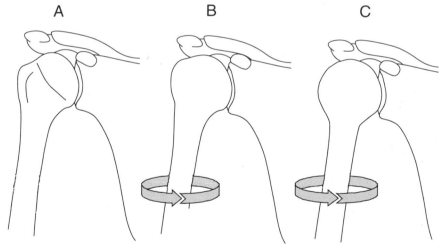

Figure 4.21. *The effect of internal rotation on the contour of the humeral head. Standard AP radiographs are always obtained with the humerus positioned with slight external rotation and this accounts for the humeral head looking like a walking stick* **(a)**. *But in the absence of any dislocation or subluxation the joint may be so painful that the arm is held in internal rotation. When this occurs then a light-bulb appearance* **(b, c)** *results and this can mimic a posterior dislocation.*

Acromio-clavicular (A-C) joint subluxation and dislocation

■ Evaluate this joint on the AP view only. The Y view can be misleading.

■ The width of the normal joint is very variable but is less than 10 mm in adults.

■ On the AP view the *inferior* surfaces of the acromion and clavicle should be in a straight line (Fig. 4.22).

■ Subluxation is detected as a step between the inferior surfaces of the acromion and the clavicle (Fig. 4.23).

■ Sometimes the appearance will be equivocal. In these cases joint separation will be revealed if a radiograph is obtained whilst the patient holds a weight in each hand. This allows comparison between the injured and uninjured sides.

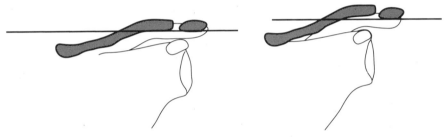

Figure 4.22. *Normal and abnormal alignment of the inferior surfaces of the acromion and the clavicle. Normal on the left, subluxation on the right.*

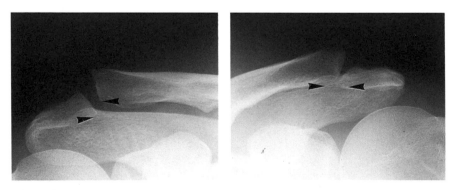

Figure 4.23. *AP radiograph of both shoulders obtained with a weight held in each hand. Normal alignment of the left A–C joint, subluxation of the right A–C joint.*

KEY POINTS

■ Obtain and scrutinize two views:

'*assessing one view only is one view too few*'.

■ Understand the normal anatomy on the second view.

■ Anterior dislocation. Diagnosis is easy. Always request a post-reduction film.

■ Posterior dislocation. Frequently missed. Diagnosis is easy when the normal anatomy on the second view is understood.

■ Acromio-clavicular joint. The inferior aspects of the acromion and clavicle should be in a straight line on the AP view.

References

1. Garth WP, Slappey CE, Ochs CW. Roentgenographic demonstration of instability of the shoulder: The apical oblique projection. *J Bone Joint Surg* 1984, **66A:** 1450–1453.
2. Wallace W, Hellier M. Improving radiographs of the injured shoulder. *Radiography* 1983, **49:** 229–232.

5 ELBOW

BASIC RADIOGRAPHS

- AP.
- lateral.

IMPORTANT ANATOMY

On the AP view:

- The olecranon is hidden.
- The capitellum articulates with the radial head – which is lateral.
- The trochlea articulates with the ulna – which is medial.

On the lateral view:

- The capitellum and trochlea are superimposed.
- There are two pads of fat. These are situated anterior and posterior to the distal humerus, and are in contact with the joint capsule. Fat is seen as a black streak in the surrounding grey soft tissues.
- In normal patients the posterior fat pad is never visible, but the anterior fat pad may be seen closely applied to the humerus (Fig. 5.1).

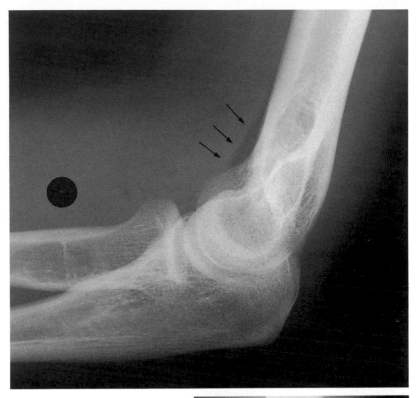

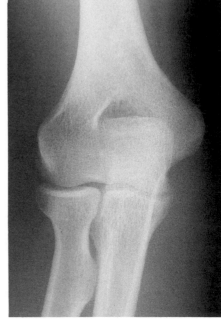

Figure 5.1. *Normal AP and lateral radiographs. A normally positioned anterior fat pad is seen as slightly darker than the surrounding muscle (arrows). This normal anterior fat pad is also well shown in Fig. 5.13 (5).*

INJURIES

■ Most fractures are readily identified.

■ A few fractures are not easy to see. Look for:

　▨ fat pad displacement;

　▨ an abnormal anterior humeral line;

　▨ an abnormal radio-capitellar line.

■ **In children**, also look for displacement of the ossification centre for the internal epicondyle.

Fat pad displacement

■ When an effusion is present it displaces the fat pads away from the bone (Fig. 5.2).

■ A visible posterior fat pad is always abnormal (Fig. 5.3).

■ A visible anterior fat pad may be normal, but if *displaced* anteriorly is abnormal.

■ If there is displacement of either of these fat pads assume that a fracture is present *whether or not a fracture can be seen.*

■ Absence of a visible fat pad does not exclude a fracture.

■ Fat pad displacement, but no obvious fracture. Look carefully for a:

　▨ radial head fracture;

　▨ supracondylar fracture of the humerus, particularly in children.

■ Fat pad displacement, and the bones still appear normal.

　▨ Do not request any additional radiographs.

　▨ Treat as for a radial head fracture.

　▨ Review in 10 days:

　　❏ if clinically normal: no further radiography;

　　❏ if clinically abnormal: obtain repeat views (Fig. 5.4).

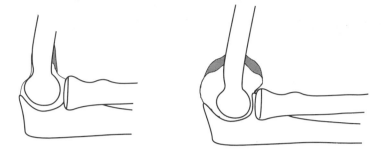

Figure 5.2. *Position of the normal anterior fad pad (left). A joint effusion displaces the anterior and posterior fat pads away from the humerus (right).*

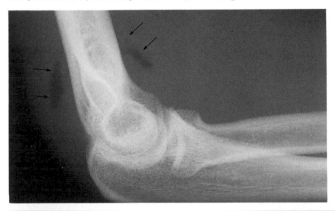

Figure 5.3. *An effusion displaces the anterior and posterior fat pads (arrows).*

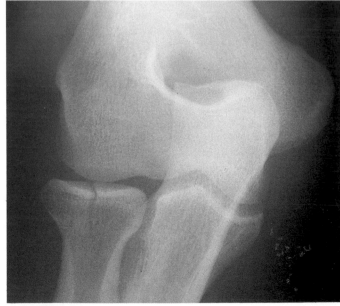

Figure 5.4. *An earlier lateral film showed displacement of the fat pads, but a fracture was not identified. This radiograph was obtained a few days later. The fracture of the radial head is now clearly visible.*

Abnormal anterior humeral line

■ **On a good lateral film** a line can be traced along the anterior cortex of the humerus. In most patients approximately one third of the capitellum lies anterior to this line (Fig. 5.5).

■ **If less than one third of the capitellum** lies anterior to this line then there may be a supracondylar fracture with the distal fragment displaced posteriorly (Fig. 5.6).

(a)   (b)

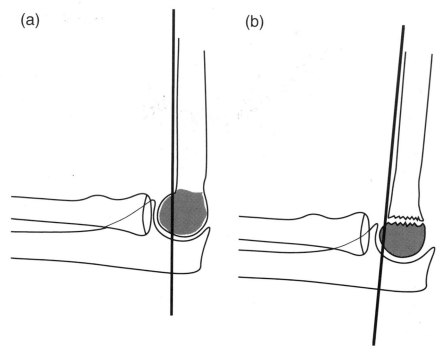

Figure 5.5. *The anterior humeral line.* **(a)** *Normal and* **(b)** *abnormal. In most normal patients approximately one third of the capitellum (shaded) lies anterior to this line. With a supracondylar fracture the distal fragment is sometimes displaced posteriorly and as a consequence less than one third of the capitellum lies anterior to the line* **(b)**.

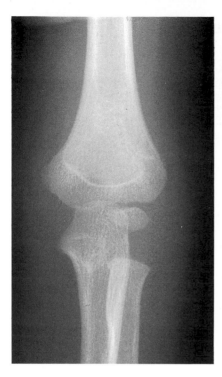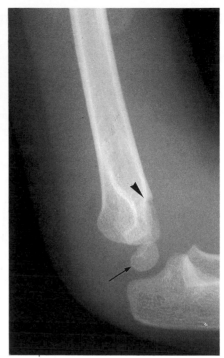

Figure 5.6. *Anterior humeral line. The AP view on the left is normal. When the lateral view was assessed it was noted that the anterior humeral line did not have a third of the capitellum (arrow) in front of it. This led to further evaluation of both the AP and lateral films and the supracondylar fracture (arrowhead) was identified. Note the displaced posterior fat pad.*

Pitfall: This rule does not apply to all patients. It is not always reliable in very young children particularly when there is only partial ossification of the capitellum. If the anterior humeral line appears abnormal then it is worth seeking another opinion.

Abnormal radiocapitellar line

■ A line drawn along the centre of the shaft of the proximal radius should pass through the capitellum (Figs 5.7 and 5.8).

■ If this line does not pass through the capitellum then a dislocation of the radial head is probable.

■ This rule is **always** valid on a true lateral film (Figs 5.9 and 5.10).

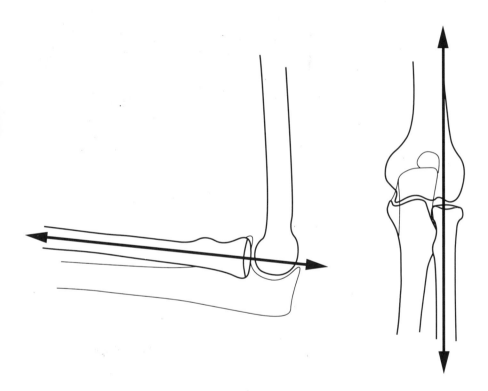

Figure 5.7. *Normal radiocapitellar line on the AP and lateral views.*

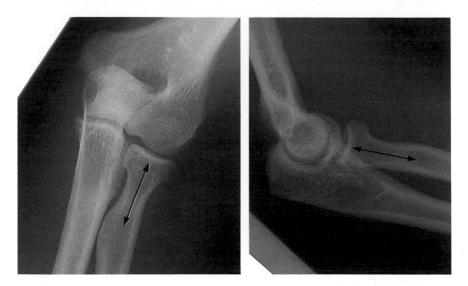

Figure 5.8. *The normal radiocapitellar line. Note: on the AP view (left) the line is drawn along the centre of the proximal portion of the radius.*

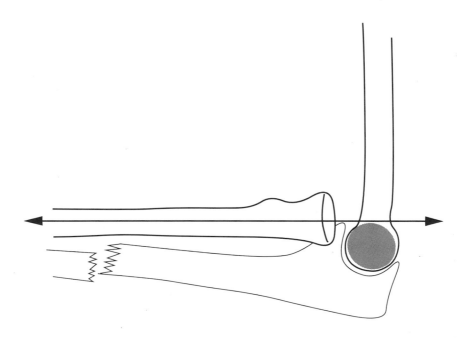

Figure 5.9. *Abnormal radiocapitellar line. On the lateral view the line does not pass through the capitellum (shaded). This indicates that the head of the radius is dislocated.*

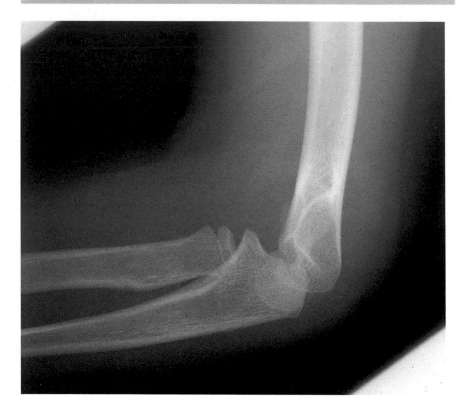

Figure 5.10. *The radiocapitellar line does not pass through the Capitellum. This indicates that the radial head is dislocated in relation to the capitellum. (In this patient the abnormal alignment is the result of a dislocation of the entire elbow joint.)*

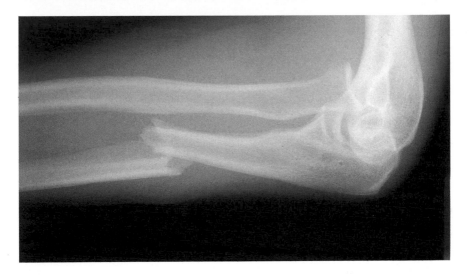

Figure 5.11. *Fracture of the shaft of the ulna with overlap of fragments. There is an associated dislocation of the radial head which is identifed by drawing the radio capitellar line. This injury is known as a Monteggia fracture dislocation.*

Pitfall: On some AP views a false impression of a dislocated radius may be suggested because this line appears abnormal. This is usually due to difficulty in obtaining an optimum position during radiography. If this rule is broken on either the AP or lateral view a second opinion should be sought.

Pitfall: The radiocapitellar line should always be drawn whenever there is a fracture of the shaft of the ulna. There may be an associated dislocation of the radial head. This is known as a Monteggia fracture dislocation (Fig. 5.11).

Children - Ossification centres

■ At birth, the ends of the radius, ulna and humerus are present only as lumps of cartilage which are not visible on the x-ray film. The large gap between the distal humerus and the proximal radius and ulna is normal.

■ During childhood, six separate ossification centres (Fig. 5.12) appear at various intervals (six months to 12 years). Four of these centres belong to the humerus, one to the radius, and one to the ulna (Fig. 5.13). The four humeral centres ossify, enlarge, coalesce and eventually fuse to the shaft.

■ The age at which each ossification centre appears is not important.

■ The sequence (Fig. 5.13) in which the centres ossify *is important.*

■ The acronym **CRITOL** gives the most common order in which the centres appear on the radiograph:

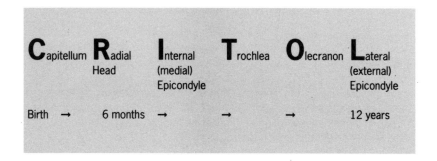

Why the CRITOL sequence is important – avulsion of the internal epicondyle

■ The ossification centre for the internal epicondyle is the point of attachment of the forearm flexor muscles. Muscular contraction may avulse this centre (Fig. 5.14). Paradoxically, minor displacement (Fig. 5.15) is often more obvious than major displacement. The internal epicondyle may come to lie within the joint. When this occurs, the detached epicondyle may be misinterpreted as being one of the other normal ossification centres (Fig. 5.16).

■ Though the **CRITOL** sequence does not occur in all patients, the trochlear centre invariably ossifies after the internal epicondyle. **If the trochlea is seen then there must be an ossified internal epicondyle somewhere on the radiograph.**

The CRITOL rule

■ **The question to ask:**	■ *Where is the internal epicondyle?*
■ **The rule to apply:**	■ *If the trochlear centre is seen but the internal epicondyle is not – then suspect avulsion of the epicondyle (Fig. 5.16)*

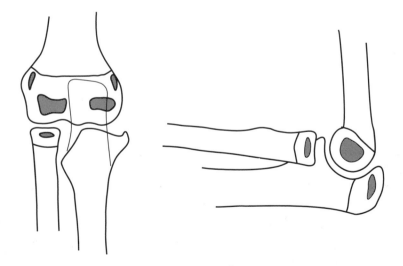

Figure 5.12. *The normal ossification centres (shaded) situated within the cartilaginous ends of the long bones.*

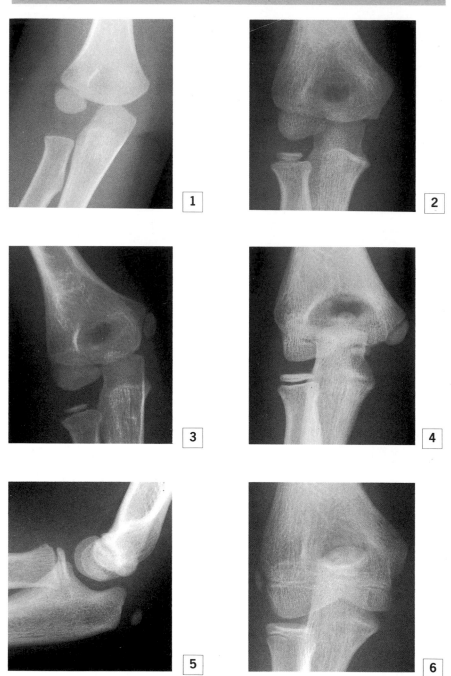

Figure 5.13. *The sequence (1–6) in which the ossification centres usually appear on the radiograph.* **CRITOL**.

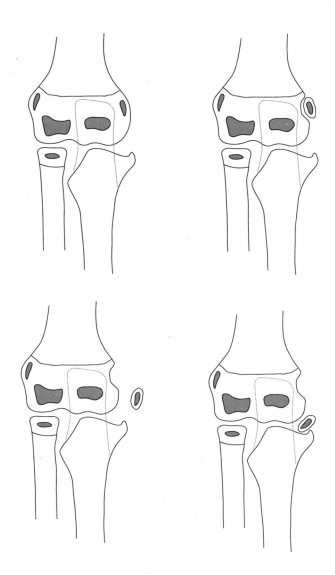

Figure 5.14. *Avulsion of the internal epicondyle.*

Figure 5.15. *Minor displacement of the internal epicondyle.*

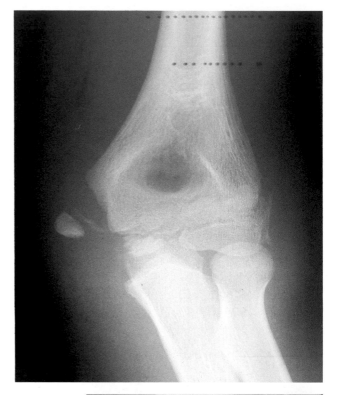

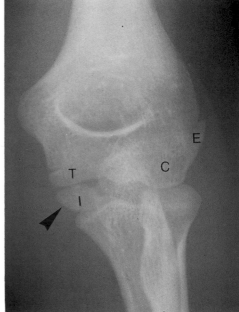

Figure 5.16. *Major displacement of the internal epicondyle. It is situated within the elbow joint (arrow head). (C = capitellum; I = internal epicondyle; T = trochlea; E = external (lateral) epicondyle.)*

KEY POINTS

■ A visible anterior fat pad is normal, but *displacement* of the anterior fat pad raises the strong probability of a fracture.

■ A visible posterior fat pad is always abnormal. A fracture is probable.

■ Absence of a displaced fat pad does not exclude a fracture.

■ The sequence in which the secondary centres usually ossify: **CRITOL**.

■ **'I before T'**. The trochlear epiphysis does not ossify before the internal epicondyle.

■ **Anterior humeral line**...what is its relation to the capitellum? In most normal elbows a third or more of the capitellum will be anterior to this line.

■ **Radio-capitellar line**...does a line drawn along the the centre of the shaft of the radius pass through the centre of the capitellum on the lateral film? If not, a dislocated head of the radius is probable.

■ **The internal epicondyle**...is it in the joint, mistaken for the trochlear ossification centre?

6 WRIST AND DISTAL FOREARM

BASIC RADIOGRAPHS

- PA.
- Lateral.

IMPORTANT ANATOMY

On the PA view:

- The carpal bones (Figs 6.1 and 6.2) are arranged in two rows. Strong ligaments bind the bones together.
- The joint spaces are uniform in width; 1–2 mm wide in the adult.

On the lateral view:

- Bony alignment may seem confusing, but the important anatomy is actually very simple to identify (Fig. 6.3):
  - *the radius, the lunate and the capitate articulate with each other and lie in a straight line. Like an apple in a cup on a saucer (Fig. 6.4).*
  - *the capitate (the apple) sits in the concavity of the lunate (the cup) which sits on the radius (the saucer).*

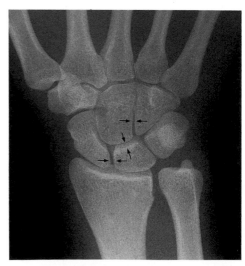

Figure 6.1. *PA radiograph. Normal wrist. Note: the spaces between the carpal bones are uniform in size (arrows).*

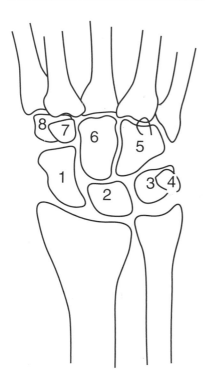

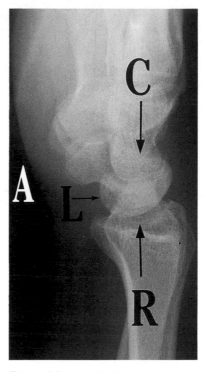

Figure 6.2. 1, scaphoid (navicular); 2, lunate; 3, triquetral; 4, pisiform; 5, hamate; 6, capitate; 7, trapezoid (lesser multangular); 8, trapezium (greater multangular).

Figure 6.3. Lateral radiograph. Normal wrist. The important relationships are between the radius (R), the lunate (L), and the capitate (C), A = Anterior.

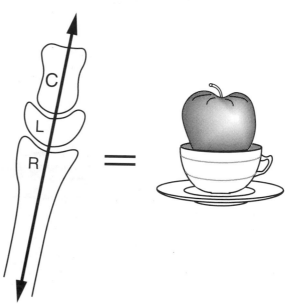

Figure 6.4. Lateral wrist. The radius, lunate and capitate lie in a straight line.

INJURIES

Fractures – distal radius

Usually easy to detect:

■ Posterior displacement of the distal fragment = Colles'.

■ Anterior displacement of the distal fragment = Smith's.

■ Greenstick (see page 228).

More difficult to detect:

■ A longitudinal fracture extending to the joint surface (Fig. 6.5).

■ A subtle break in the cortex over the dorsal aspect of the distal radius (Fig. 6.6).

■ An impacted undisplaced fracture. The only abnormality may be a very slight increase in bone density (Fig. 6.7).

■ A slight ripple in the cortex. A torus fracture (Fig. 6.8). This is a very common injury in children.

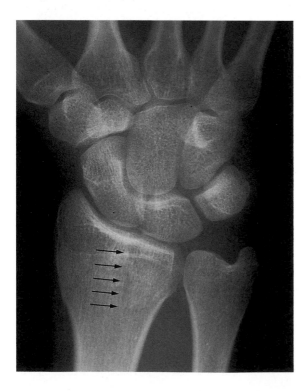

Figure 6.5. *Longitudinal fracture of the distal radius extending to the articular surface.*

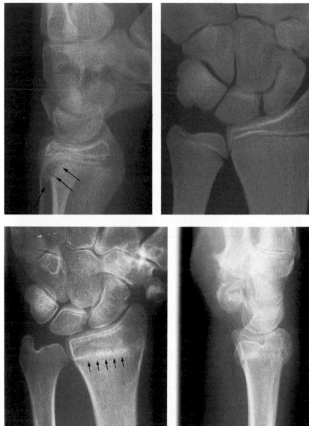

Figure 6.6. *Subtle fracture of the distal radius seen only on the lateral view.*

Figure 6.7. *An impacted undisplaced fracture of the distal radius is shown only as a white (sclerotic) line.*

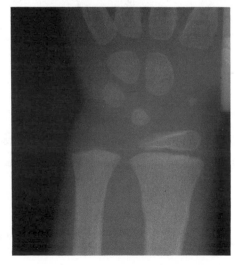

Figure 6.8. *Torus fracture. Identified by the slight bulge in the radial cortex.*

Fractures – scaphoid

- If there is 'snuff box' tenderness, scaphoid views should be requested (Fig. 6.9). The particular views vary between hospitals but it is common practice to have a standard set of at least four different projections. Some fractures are very difficult to demonstrate (Figs 6.10 and 6.11).

- Fractures across the waist of the bone jeopardize the blood supply of the proximal fragment. If the patient is managed incorrectly then non-union, delayed union or avascular necrosis may result.

Site of fracture	Incidence	Risk of avascular necrosis
Waist	80%	+++
Proximal pole	10%	++++
Distal pole (Fig. 6.12)	10%	0

- If scaphoid views have been obtained following an acute injury, it is mandatory that the patient is followed up, whether or not a fracture has been demonstrated. There are no exceptions to this rule. Some scaphoid fractures are not detectable until 5–10 days after the injury. Resorption of bone around the fracture has usually occurred by then and most fractures become obvious.

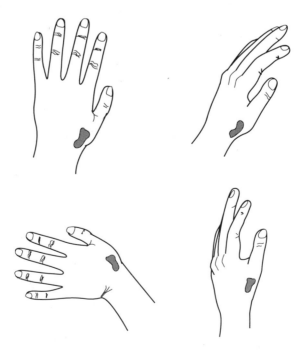

Figure 6.9. *Scaphoid fractures are often very difficult to identify, and it is common for four views to be obtained.*

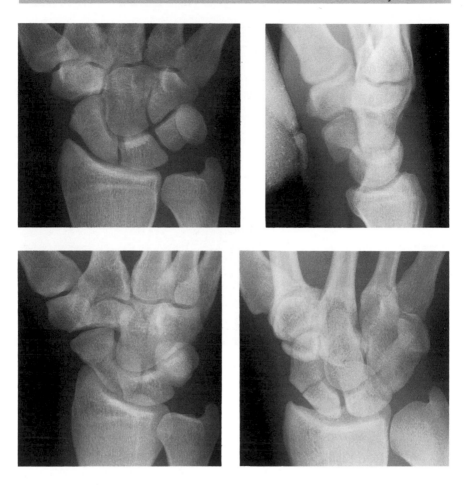

Figure 6.10. *Scaphoid fracture seen on one view only.*

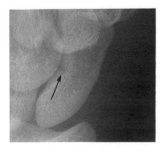

Figure 6.11. *This subtle fracture through the waist of the scaphoid was identifiable on one view only.*

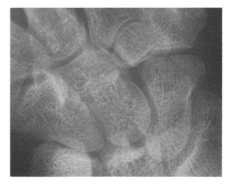

Figure 6.12. *Fracture through the distal pole of the scaphoid.*

Other fractures of the carpal bones

- Are rare; 90% of carpal bone fractures are through the scaphoid.

- Occasionally, a small fragment may be seen lying posterior to the proximal row of carpal bones on the lateral view. This is usually a fracture of the triquetrum (Fig. 6.13).

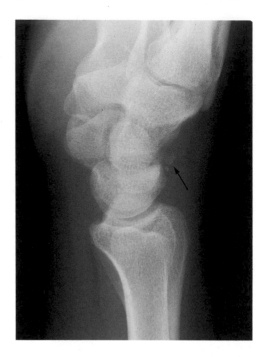

Figure 6.13. *Two small bone fragments lie posterior to the carpus. Their origin cannot be clearly identified. A fragment in this position on the lateral view usually represents a triquetral fracture.*

Lunate dislocation

- Most dislocations involve the lunate bone. All other dislocations are exceptionally rare.

- The important radiograph is the lateral. Recognition of a dislocation is not difficult provided the normal anatomy on the lateral view is understood (Figs 6.3 and 6.4). The distal radius, the lunate and the capitate articulate with each other and lie in a straight line.

'The capitate sits in the concavity of the lunate'

Radiological features:

- The lunate dislocates anteriorly.

- *The concavity of the lunate is empty* on the lateral view (Fig. 6.14).

- The radius and the capitate remain in a straight line on the lateral view (Fig. 6.15).

- It is commonly emphasized that on the PA view a dislocated lunate adopts a triangular configuration instead of its normal 'squarish' contour. Although this sign can be helpful, **it is much easier to recognize a dislocation by scrutinizing the lateral view** (Fig. 6.15).

Figure 6.14. *Lunate dislocation. The PA view shows that the lunate appears triangular (arrowed). Compare this with the normal appearance seen in Fig. 6.1.*

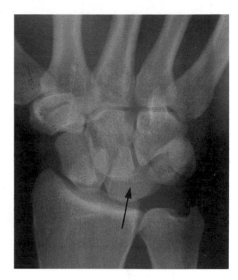

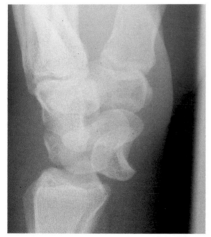

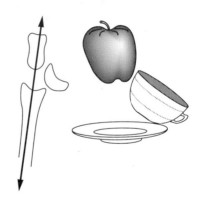

Figure 6.15. *Lunate dislocation. Lateral radiograph showing the lunate dislocated anteriorly. The concavity of the lunate ('the cup') is empty. The radius and capitate remain in a straight line.*

Perilunate dislocation

■ The whole of the carpus (except for the lunate) is displaced posteriorly.

■ Inspection of the lateral view will reveal the malalignment of the carpal bones (Fig. 6.16).

■ *Once again, the concavity of the lunate is empty.* In this instance the radius and lunate remain in a straight line. The capitate lies posteriorly and out of line.

■ A perilunate dislocation is often associated with a scaphoid fracture (Fig. 6.17), an injury known as a trans scapho-perilunate dislocation.

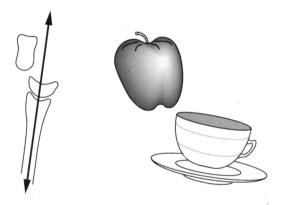

Figure 6.16. *Perilunate dislocation. The capitate is displaced posteriorly. The concavity of the lunate ('the cup') is empty. The radius and the lunate remain in a straight line.*

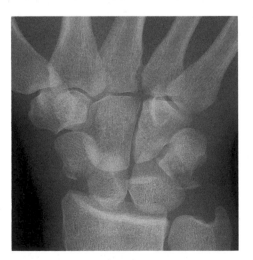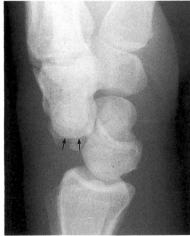

Figure 6.17. *Perilunate dislocation. The concavity of the lunate is empty. The capitate (arrows) is displaced posteriorly. (There are also associated fractures of the scaphoid and triquetrum).*

Carpal subluxations

■ Ligamentous rupture at any of the small joints of the carpus can occur. This may result in carpal instability and cause pain or reduced function.

■ The joint spaces between the intercarpal joints should measure no more than 2 mm in the adult. Widening of any of these spaces (Figs 6.18 and 6.19) raises the possibility of an intercarpal subluxation. Referral to a hand surgeon will be necessary.

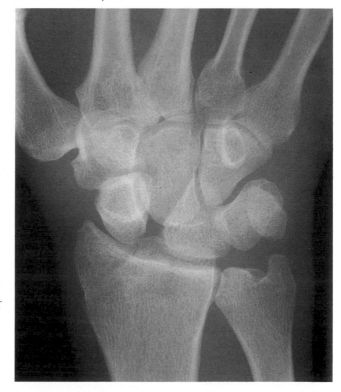

Figure 6.18. (a) *normal PA view.* **(b)** *shows widening of the joint space (shaded area) between the scaphoid and the lunate. This indicates a ligamentous injury.*

Figure 6.19. *Zone of vulnerability. Fracture through the radial styloid process. Note also the abnormal widening of the joint between the scaphoid and the lunate bones which indicates severe ligamentous disruption. (The lateral view would also need to be scrutinized so as to evaluate the alignment between the radius, lunate and capitate.)*

Combination injuries

■ Injuries of the wrist and carpus are not always solitary. They may occur as various combinations of the fractures and dislocations described above.

■ The concept of a *zone of vulnerability* at the wrist is helpful in identifying combination injuries.

　▢ The zone (Fig. 6.20) passes through the radial styloid process, the scaphoid, the proximal parts of the capitate and hamate, the triquetral and the ulnar styloid process.

　▢ If an abnormality is identified within this arc careful scrutiny should be made for additional fractures or dislocations (Figs 6.17 and 6.19).

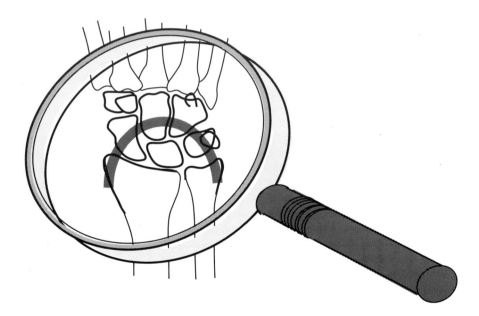

Figure 6.20. *The zone of vulnerability (shaded). If one abnormality is detected within this area, then it is important to look for other injuries elsewhere in the zone.*

KEY POINTS

■ Clinical examination determines the appropriate views:

▓ a wrist series;

or

▓ a scaphoid series.

■ A request for a scaphoid series means that the patient must be followed up – *even if the radiographs appear normal.*

■ Inspection of the lateral view is very important. It may be the *only* view which shows:

▓ a break in the posterior cortex of the radius

▓ a torus fracture

▓ a carpal dislocation

■ The most common carpal dislocations (lunate or perilunate) are readily diagnosed from the lateral view. Apply the simple rule:

'The concavity of the lunate should never be empty'

■ Any of the intercarpal ligaments may tear and cause instability and pain. If an intercarpal joint measures more than 2 mm in an adult – suspect a ligamentous injury.

7 HANDS AND FINGERS

Some seemingly minor fractures involving the digits may have important clinical implications and these can often be deduced from the radiographic findings. If the significance of the radiological appearances are not appreciated then subsequent management may be inappropriate.

BASIC RADIOGRAPHS

Precise clinical information indicating the site of injury will ensure that the most suitable radiographic projections are obtained, as follows:

■ Injuries to the metacarpals or phalanges – PA and oblique projections of the entire hand.

■ Single finger or thumb injuries – PA and lateral projections of the digit.

IMPORTANT ANATOMY

Carpo-metacarpal joints

■ On the PA view of the hand (Fig. 7.1) the spaces comprising the carpo-metacarpal joints are identifiable and approximately equal (1–2 mm). This is the same as the space between the carpal bones (see Chapter 6).

■ When a carpo-metacarpal dislocation is present this space may be obliterated by the overlapping bones.

Fingers

Knowledge of the anatomical attachments of the tendons and ligaments is essential in order to appreciate the clinical significance of the radiographic appearances.

■ The collateral ligaments extend from the lateral and medial margins of each metacarpal and each phalanx, across the joint, and insert into the same margin at the base of the adjacent phalanx (Fig. 7.2).

■ The volar plate is a thickening of the joint capsule on the palmar aspect of each joint and it attaches to the base of the adjacent phalanx (Fig. 7.3).

■ The extensor tendons insert into the dorsal surfaces at the base of each phalanx (Fig. 7.3).

Figure 7.1. *Normal hand. PA view. Note that the joint spaces at the bases of the metacarpals are equal. They are the same width as the joint spaces between the carpal bones.*

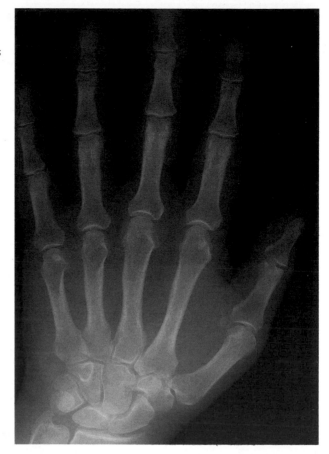

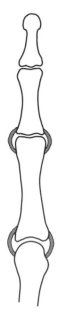

Figure 7.2. *The collateral ligaments. They are inserted into the bases of the phalanges.*

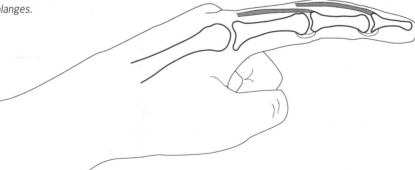

Figure 7.3. *The volar plate is a thickening of the joint capsule. It inserts into the base of the phalanx on its palmar surface. The extensor tendons insert into the bases of the phalanges on the dorsal surface.*

INJURIES

Fractures – hands and fingers

■ Most fractures involving the mid-shaft of a phalanx or a metacarpal are stable and pose few clinical problems. They are often managed by garter strapping (buddy strapping).

■ **Some fractures do require orthopaedic referral.** The following radiographic findings indicate a clinically important injury:

▨ Extension of the fracture to a joint surface (Fig. 7.4).

▨ A spiral fracture of the shaft with rotation of the fragments (Fig. 7.5). The degree of rotation needs to be assessed clinically (ref. 1).

▨ Avulsion of a bone fragment at the base of a phalanx (Table 7.1).

■ Avulsion of an extensor tendon results in a mallet finger (Fig. 7.8). The importance of clinical examination in the detection of this injury needs emphasis since **a bone fragment is present in only 25% of cases of mallet finger.** An isolated flexion deformity of the distal phalanx of a finger is almost impossible without avulsion or rupture of the extensor tendon.

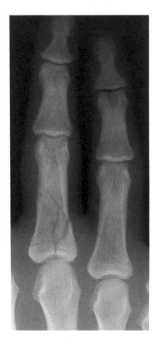

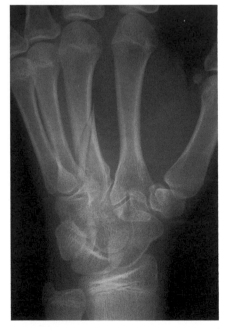

Figure 7.4. *Undisplaced fracture of the proximal phalanx. This injury is clinically important because the fracture involves the joint surface.*

Figure 7.5. *Spiral fracture of a metacarpal. The degree of rotation cannot be adequately assessed from the radiograph alone. Clinical assessment is more accurate (ref. 1).*

Table 7.1 Small fractures can be important.

Site of bone fragment	Avulsion of the:
Lateral or medial	collateral ligament (Fig.7.6)
Palmar	volar plate (Fig. 7.7)
Dorsal	extensor tendon (Fig. 7.8)

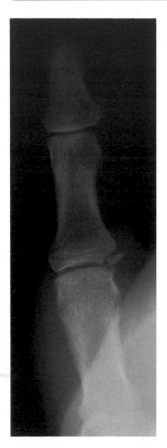 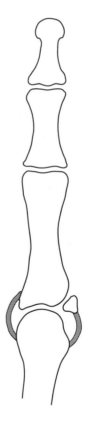

Figure 7.6. *Fracture at the base of a phalanx at the point of insertion of the medial collateral ligament.*

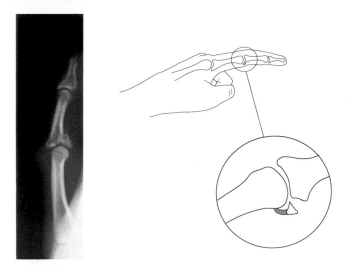

Figure 7.7. *Fracture at the base of a phalanx at the point of insertion of the volar plate.*

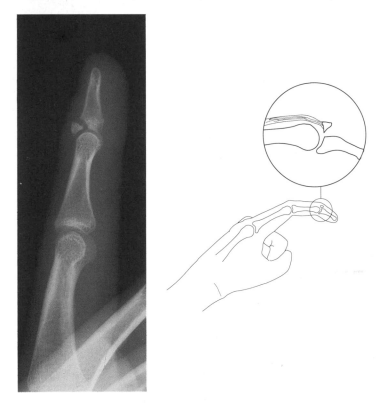

Figure 7.8. *Fracture at the base of a phalanx at the point of insertion of the extensor tendon.*

Fractures - thumb

■ **Bennett's fracture.** A fracture at the base of the first metacarpal extending into the joint surface with dislocation at the carpo-metacarpal joint (Fig. 7.9). The metacarpal is pulled dorsally and radially by the abductor pollicis longus muscle. This fracture–dislocation may require open reduction and internal fixation.

■ **Gamekeeper's thumb.** This results from a rupture of the ulnar collateral ligament (Fig. 7.10). Occasionally there may be a bone fragment at the site of the avulsion, but more frequently the bone is intact. If this injury is suspected clinically then stress radiographs may assist in confirming the diagnosis. A complete tear of the ligament requires surgical repair.

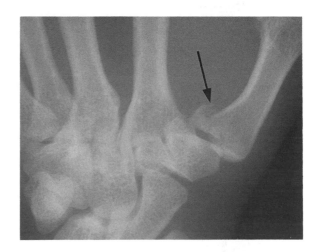

Figure 7.9. *Bennett's fracture (oblique view). The fracture at the base of the first metacarpal (arrow) involves the joint surface.*

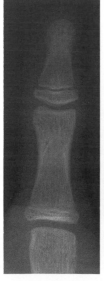

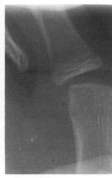

Figure 7.10. *Gamekeeper's thumb. The medial collateral ligament has been ruptured. In the neutral position no abnormality is apparent. When abduction stress is applied (right) the joint becomes abnormally wide.*

Carpo-metacarpal dislocations

These are clinically important. Note:

■ The fourth and fifth joints are those most commonly affected.

■ Dislocation is commonly associated with a fracture at the base of the metacarpal.

■ Loss of the normal joint space at the base of the metacarpal on the PA film raises the strong possibility of this injury (Fig. 7.11).

■ The oblique film usually demonstrates a dislocation most clearly.

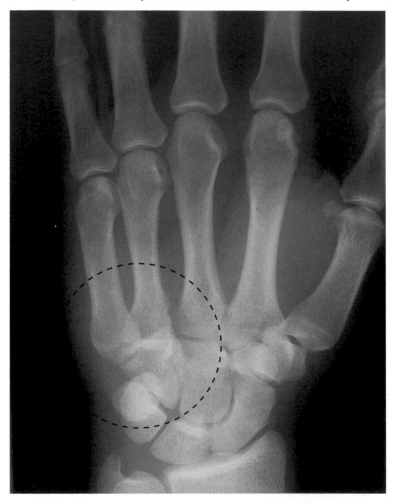

Figure 7.11. *PA view. Carpo-metacarpal dislocation. The joint spaces at the bases of the fourth and fifth metacarpals are not visualized because the dislocated bones are overlapping.*

KEY POINTS

■ Most fractures are easy to detect. Some apparently minor fractures have important implications and need an orthopaedic referral.

■ **It is important to look for small fragments of bone detached from the margin of a joint.**

■ A spiral fracture of a metacarpal with rotation of the fragments may require internal fixation. Rotation is best assessed clinically.

■ Ligamentous injuries without a fracture are common and will not show a radiographic abnormality. These injuries may be overlooked unless clinical examination is very thorough.

■ The following injuries need to be referred for specialist assessment and management:

▓ carpo-metacarpal dislocations;

▓ clinically unstable fractures;

▓ spiral fracture with rotation;

▓ fractures involving articular surfaces.

Reference

1. Green DP, Rowland SA. Fractures and dislocations in the hand. In: Rockwood CA Jr and Green DP (eds) *Fractures*. JB Lippincott, Philadelphia, 1975.

8 CERVICAL SPINE

Following trauma there is no need for radiography (refs 1, 2) in any patient who meets all of the following criteria:

- conscious;
- not intoxicated;
- no abnormal neurological findings;
- no neck pain or tenderness.

BASIC RADIOGRAPHS

- Usually 3 views are obtained:
  - long AP;
  - lateral to include the top of the T1 vertebral body;
  - open mouth AP to show the C1–C2 articulation – *(the peg view)*;
- In some centres two additional trauma obliques are also obtained (refs 3 and 4).

IMPORTANT ANATOMY

Normal lateral view
Vertebral alignment

- Three lines (or arcs) can be traced:
  1. Along the anterior margins of the vertebral bodies.
  2. Along the posterior margins of the vertebral bodies.
  3. Along the bases of the spinous processes.

- These lines (Figs 8.1 and 8.2) should be smooth unbroken arcs.
- Line 3 may sometimes show a slight step at C2, particularly in children. This posterior step (Fig. 8.3) *should not be more than 2 mm* behind the smooth arc traced from C3 to C1.

Vertebral bodies

- Those below C2 have a fairly uniform square/rectangular shape.

Intervertebral discs

■ These should be of uniform height.

Odontoid peg

■ The dens can be visualized just behind the anterior arch of the C1 vertebra. It should be closely applied to the posterior aspect of the C1 arch. The normal distance between the bones at this point is no more than 3 mm in adults and 5 mm in children (Figs 8.4 and 8.5).

Soft tissues

■ The soft tissue shadow anterior to the vertebral bodies has:

■ a characteristic configuration (Fig. 8.6);

■ standard widths (Table 8.1).

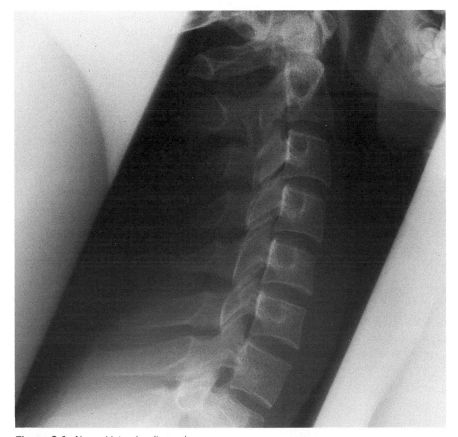

Figure 8.1. *Normal lateral radiograph.*

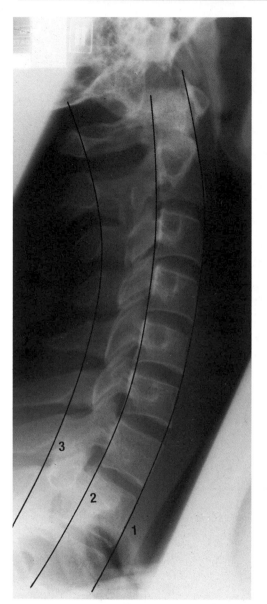

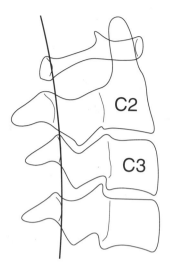

Figure 8.3. *The upper cervical vertebrae. Checking the three lines. Note: line 3 does not pass precisely along the base of the C2 spinous process. This is a normal finding provided that there is no more than a 2 mm gap between the C3–C1 line and the base of the C2 spinous process. A gap larger than 2 mm is abnormal, and may indicate a fracture or dislocation at the C2 level.*

Figure 8.2. *Normal lateral view. The three lines which need to be checked in all patients, to assess whether vertebral alignment is normal (see text).*

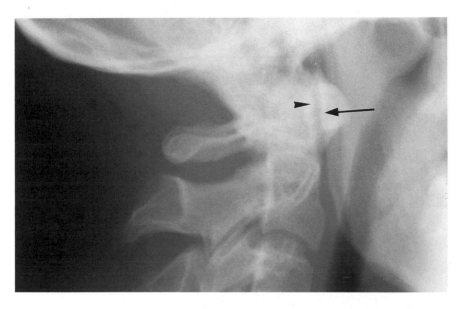

Figure 8.4. *The normal distance between the anterior arch of C1 (arrow) and the anterior aspect of the odontoid peg (arrowhead) should be no more than 3 mm in an adult.*

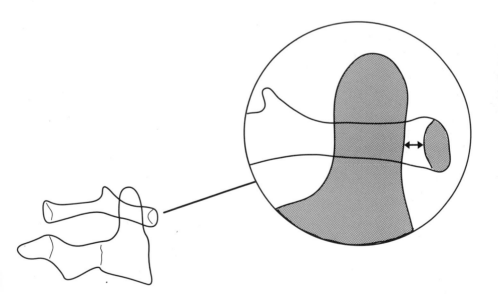

Figure 8.5. *Normal relationship between the anterior arch of C1 and the odontoid peg. The distance indicated by the arrowheads should be no more than 3 mm in adults or 5 mm in children.*

Table 8.1 Maximum normal width of the prevertebral soft tissues.

Level	Width (mm)	Approximate % of vertebral body width
C1–4	7	30%
C5–7	22	100%

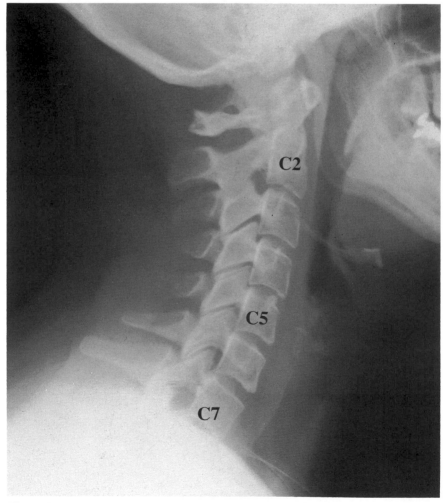

Figure 8.6. *Normal width and configuration of the soft tissues lying immediately anterior to the vertebral bodies and posterior to the airway.*

Normal long AP view

■ The spinous processes lie in a straight line (Fig. 8.7). **Exception:** This rule may appear to be broken when bifid spinous processes are present (Fig. 8.8).

■ The distance between the spinous processes should be approximately equal. No single space should be 50% wider than the one immediately above or below (ref. 5). **Exception:** This 50% rule may be broken if spasm holds the neck in flexion.

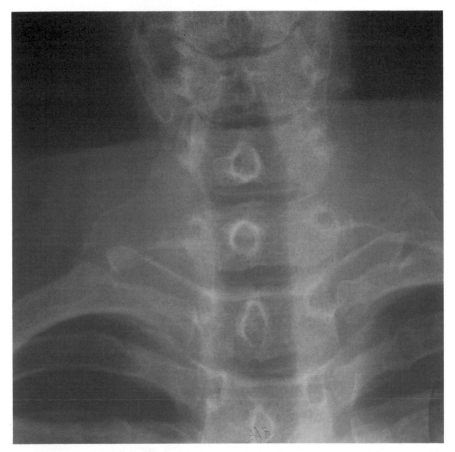

Figure 8.7. *Normal long AP view. The spinous processes lie in a straight line and are spaced equally apart.*

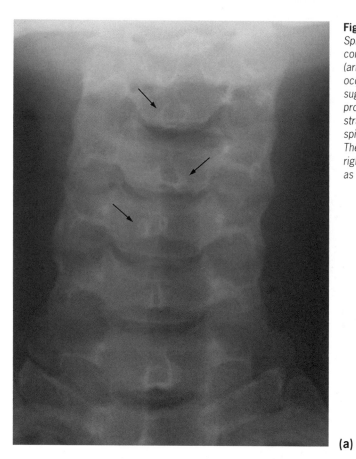

Figure 8.8. (a) *Spinous processes are commonly bifid (arrows). When this occurs it may falsely suggest that the processes are not in a straight line.* **(b)** *Bifid spinous processes. The drawing on the right shows a vertebra as viewed from above.*

(a)

(b)

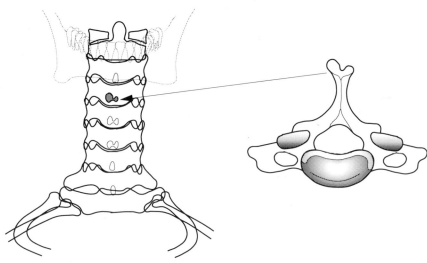

Normal AP peg view

■ The lateral margins of C1 should align with the lateral margins of C2.

■ The space on each side of the odontoid peg should be equal (Fig. 8.9 (a)). **Exception:** slight rotation of the neck may cause these spaces to appear unequal. However, if the lateral margins of C1 and C2 remain normally aligned then this asymmetry (Fig. 8.9 (b)) can be attributed to rotation.

(a)

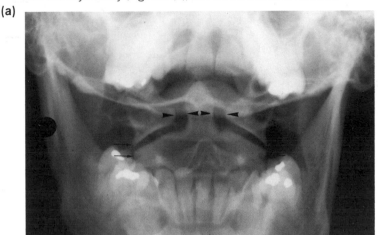

(b)

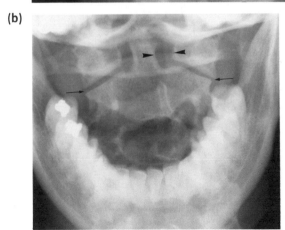

Figure 8.9. (a) *Normal AP peg view. The odontoid peg is well seen and not obscured by overlying teeth. The space on either side of the peg is equal (arrowheads). The lateral margins of C1 and C2 align (arrows).* **(b)** *An apparent abnormality due to slight rotation of the patient's neck (see text). The space (arrowheads) to the left of the odontoid peg is wider than that on the right – but the lateral margins of C1 and C2 (arrows) remain in alignment.*

INJURIES

Inspect the radiographs systematically:

Step 1. The lateral view

Injuries are most common in the lower cervical spine (C5–C7) and at the C1–C2 articulation. At least 70% of detectable abnormalities will be visible on the *lateral* radiograph (ref. 6). Inspect this view first.

1. Check that the top of T1 vertebra is seen

If the top of T1 is not demonstrated, then ask the radiographer to obtain further views (Figs 8.10 and 8.11). There are several options: a higher penetration technique, bringing the shoulders down by pulling on the arms, a 'swimmers view', or trauma obliques (refs 3, 4). All of these can be taken without moving the patient's head or neck.

2. Trace the three lines

If there is a step or kink in any of these lines then suspect a fracture or ligamentous disruption (Fig. 8.12).

3. Check the vertebral bodies

- Below C2 these should be the same size and shape.
- Any small fragment of bone may signify a fracture (Fig. 8.13).
- The spinous processes should be intact (Fig. 8.11).

4. Check the intervertebral discs

Following a very severe injury a disc space may occasionally be widened when compared with the other normal spaces above and below (ref. 8).

5. Check the soft tissues

- Look for abnormal widening (Table 8.1), or a localized bulge (Figs 8.13 and 8.14).
- Swelling of the prevertebral tissues occurs in approximately 50% of patients with a bone injury (ref. 7).
- If soft tissue swelling is present then all the views need to be scrutinized again for evidence of a bony or ligamentous injury (ref. 8).
- **Pitfall:** the absence of soft tissue swelling does not exclude a significant injury.

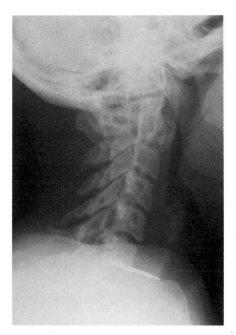 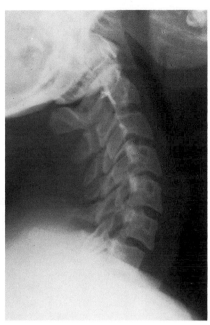

Figure 8.10. *The initial radiograph (left) appears normal. But C7 and T1 are not shown. With the shoulders pulled down (right) the forward slip of C6 on C7 is revealed. Note: this film is still not adequate. Further views must be obtained in order to show the top of T1.*

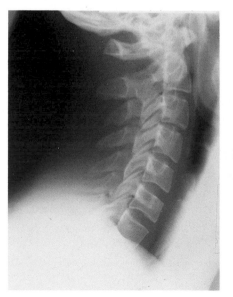 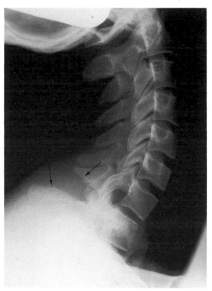

Figure 8.11. *No abnormality is seen (left). But the top of T1 vertebra has not been visualized. Subsequently the shoulders have been pulled down (right). This repeat film reveals a fracture of the spinous process of C7 (arrows) and forward subluxation of the facets of C7 on T1.*

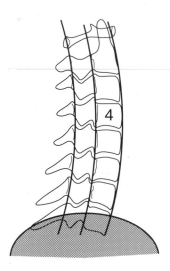 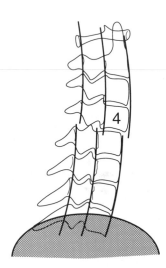

Figure 8.12. *The normal three smooth lines or arcs (left). Disruption of each of the arcs (right) indicating a forward slip of C4 on C5.*

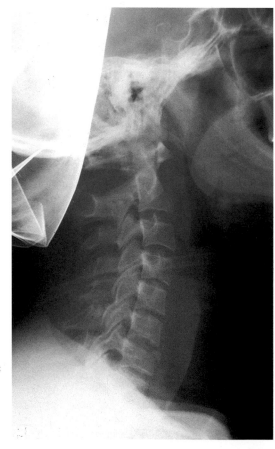

Figure 8.13. *A small bone fragment is detached from the anterior aspect of C7. Although this may appear to be a minor injury it can be associated with major ligamentous rupture and instability. Note: there is soft tissue swelling anterior to the fracture.*

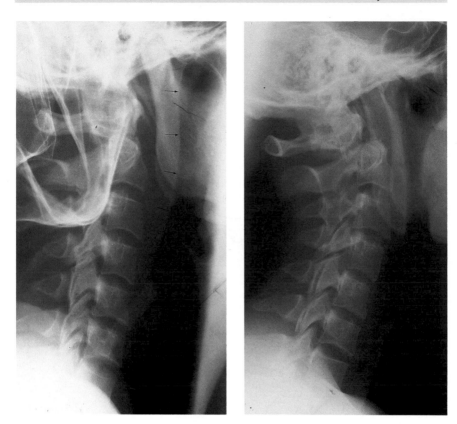

Figure 8.14. *The importance of soft tissue swelling. No bony injury is visible (left). Alignment, as indicated by the three lines is normal. The only abnormality is extensive soft tissue swelling (arrows). A repeat film two days later (right) shows a fracture at the base of the odontoid peg with marked malalignment of all three lines.*

Step 2. The long AP view

■ The spinous processes should be in a straight line. Deviation from this line may indicate a unilateral facet joint subluxation (Figs 8.15 and 8.16), If deviation is detected, scrutinize the lateral view very carefully.

■ The distances between the tips of the spinous processes should be roughly equal. Abnormal widening of an interspinous distance (Figs 8.17 and 8.18) compared with the spaces immediately above **and** below is diagnostic of an anterior cervical dislocation (ref. 5). This observation is most useful in the severely injured patient whose shoulders have obscured some of the vertebrae on the lateral view (ref. 8). Abnormal widening is an important warning that the neck must be immobilized whilst an adequate lateral view is obtained.

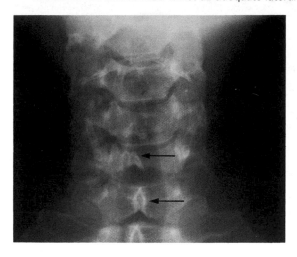

Figure 8.15. *The spinous processes (arrows) are not in line. This appearance can result from a unilateral facet joint dislocation.*

Figure 8.16.
Diagrammatic representation of a unilateral facet joint dislocation. The spinous processes do not lie in a straight line. A unilateral facet joint dislocation causes one vertebra to rotate on another. The injury as seen from above (right).

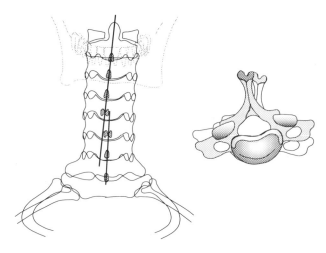

Figure 8.17. *AP view. There is abnormal widening of the space between the spinous processes (the two lower arrowheads) indicating that an anterior cervical dislocation may be present.*

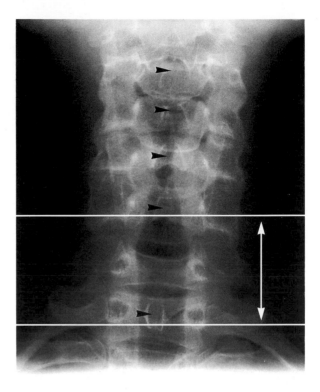

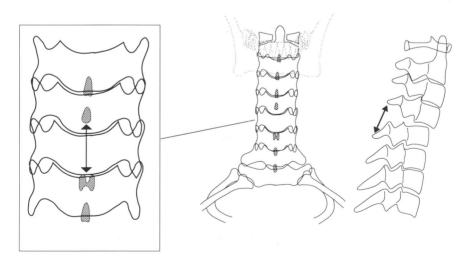

Figure 8.18. *AP view. Widening of an interspinous distance (double headed arrow). This distance is 50% greater than the spaces immediately above **and** below. This finding (ref. 5) indicates an anterior cervical dislocation (right).*

Step 3. The C1–C2 articulation

Scrutinize the atlanto-axial articulation, **using both the lateral and the peg views together:**

■ **On the lateral view look for:**

▥ Evidence of prevertebral soft tissue swelling (Fig 8.14).

▥ A fracture of the odontoid peg (Fig 8.14).

▥ A fracture of the laminae of C1 or C2 (Fig 8.19).

▥ Displacement of the posterior arch of C1 from its expected alignment along the smooth curve of line 3 – the spinolaminar line or arc (Fig. 8.20).

▥ Widening of the distance (Fig. 8.20) between the anterior margin of the peg and the posterior aspect of the arch of C1.

■ **On the open mouth 'peg' view look for:**

▥ A fracture of the odontoid peg.

Pitfall: Several artefacts mimic transverse and vertical fractures of the peg (Figs 8.21 and 8.22). These are due to superimposition of the arch of C1, the incisor teeth, the occiput, or the soft tissues at the nape of the neck (ref. 9). It is common to see a thin black line (Fig. 8.22) across the base of the peg which does **not** represent a fracture but results from the overlapping shadows from structures of different radiographic density. This optical illusion is known as a Mach band or Mach effect (ref. 11). It is important to be aware of these lines, but it is even more important to seek advice before too readily dismissing any line as an artefact.

▥ The lateral masses of C1 overhanging the lateral margins of C2 (Fig. 8.23).

▥ Unequal or asymmetrical spaces between the odontoid peg and the lateral masses of C1 (Fig. 8.23).

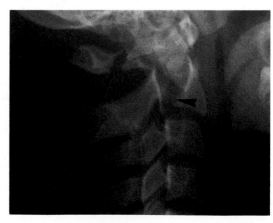

Figure 8.19. *A fracture (Hangman's fracture) of the body of C2 (arrowhead). There is also a fracture through the laminae of C1 (arrow).*

Figure 8.20. *Adult. There is abnormal widening of the space (arrowheads) between the odontoid peg and the arch of C1 (normal = 3 mm) indicating a rupture of the transverse ligament. Note: line three (the spino-laminar line) is also abnormal and the posterior arch of C1 (arrow) is displaced anteriorly.*

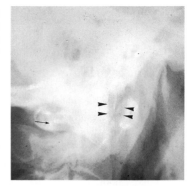

Figure 8.21. *Appearances mimicking fractures of the odontoid peg due to overlapping teeth (left), and overlap by the C1 arch (right).*

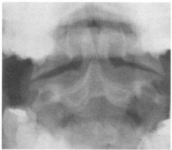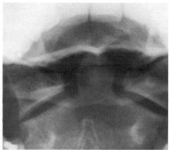

Figure 8.22. *A thin black line (arrows) crosses the base of the odontoid peg and mimics a fracture. However, it extends beyond the bone on each side. This artefact (a Mach band) is due to an optical effect resulting from overlap of structures of different radiographic density (ref. 11).*

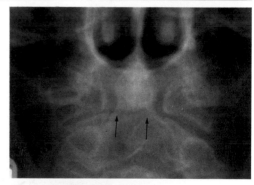

Figure 8.23. *Burst fracture of C1 (Jefferson fracture). The space on each side of the odontoid peg is widened (arrows). The lateral margins of C1 overhang those of C2 (arrowheads).*

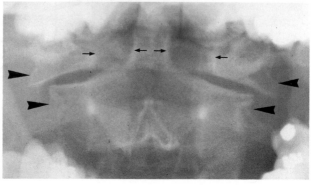

PITFALLS

Cervical spondylosis

Spondylotic changes are common over the age of 40. Distinguishing between the appearances due to spondylosis and those resulting from an acute injury is not always easy. Fortunately correlation of the clinical symptoms and signs with the site of the radiographic abnormality will provide reassurance in most instances. In other cases a conservative approach to management will be necessary until an experienced observer has reviewed the radiographs. Two effects resulting from degenerative change are:

- The smooth unbroken line along the anterior margin of the vertebral bodies may show a step (Fig. 8.24). This step is usually due to an osteophyte and may be misinterpreted as vertebral subluxation.

- There may be genuine anterior subluxation (Fig. 8.25) resulting from degenerative changes in the facet joints. There is no simple way of distinguishing this from traumatic subluxation. A cautious approach to management will be necessary.

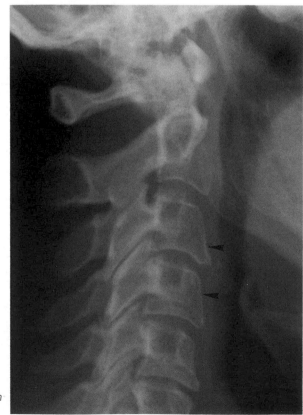

Figure 8.24. *Degenerative change. A step may occur in the smooth arc (line one) which extends along the anterior margin of the vertebral bodies. In this example the step is due to anterior osteophyte formation at the inferior margin of C3.*

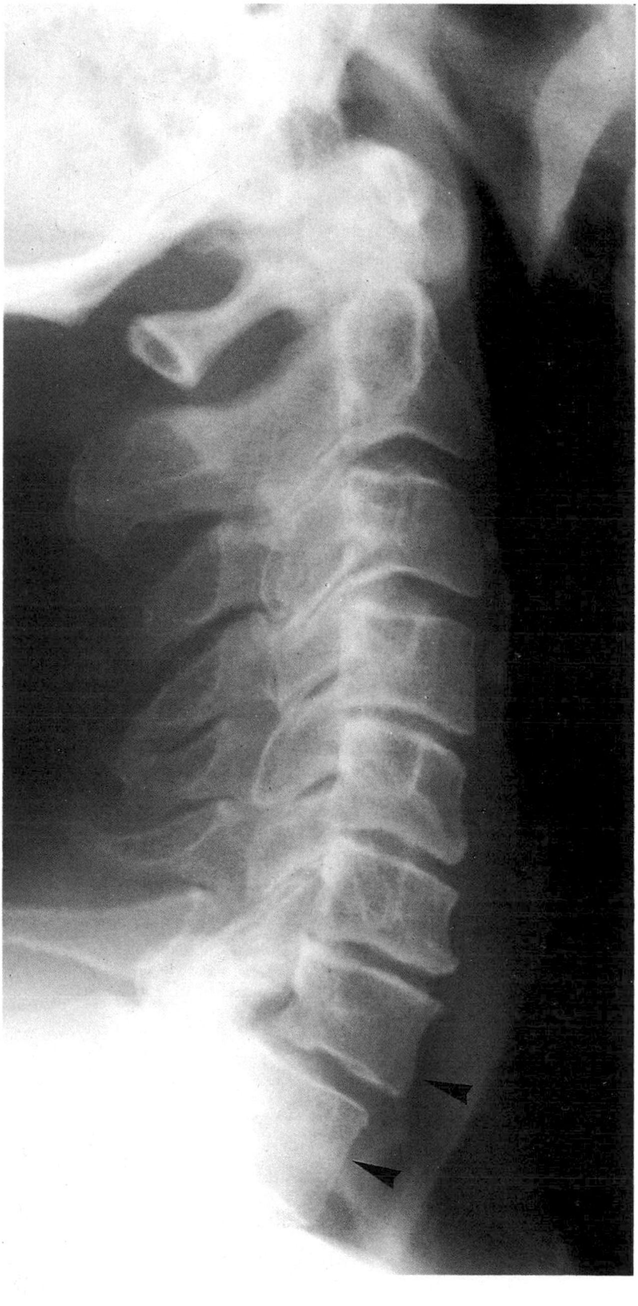

Figure 8.25.
*Degenerative change.
There is forward
subluxation of the body
of C7 on T1. This
appearance is
radiologically
indistinguishable from
a traumatic
subluxation.*

Developmental variants

■ A vertebra may appear slightly narrow anteriorly without the normal square/rectangular outline (Fig. 8.26 (a)). This may be mistaken for a compression fracture. Though this narrowing is sometimes due to old trauma it can be due to persistence of the normal slightly wedged shape which is present during adolescence (ref. 9).

■ A small calcified opacity may be present anteriorly (Fig. 8.26 (b)). This may be mistaken for a small fracture fragment. Sometimes this represents a detached osteophyte from a previous minor injury. Alternatively, it may be a remnant of an ununited secondary ossification centre of the adjacent vertebral body (ref. 9).

■ Distinguishing these appearances from an acute injury can be difficult. Sometimes the importance of the finding will depend not only on clinical correlation, but also on the intuition of an experienced observer.

a)

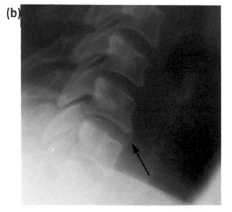

Figure 8.26. (a) *Developmental variant. The anterior aspect of a vertebral body (arrow) may appear slightly flattened. In this instance it is due to a persistence of the normal wedge shaped configuration which is commonly present during adolescence. Distinguishing this appearance from a fracture may be difficult.* (b) *Developmental variant. Calcification close to the anterior longitudinal ligament may mimic a fracture fragment. This appearance is often due to a persistent unfused secondary ossification centre belonging to the adjacent vertebral body.*

Delayed instability

■ Severe pain and spasm may make it difficult to exclude a significant injury to the posterior ligament complex. Muscle spasm can hold the neck in an anatomical position thus masking ligamentous rupture. Instability may only become evident when the spasm has resolved.

■ For this reason it is important that any patient who has severe pain and spasm, but appears fit for discharge is put in a collar and asked to re-attend within a few days for lateral views in flexion and extension. These radiographs must be taken under close clinical supervision.

■ If these additional plain films are equivocal, then it will often be necessary to refer the patient for magnetic resonance imaging (MRI), to exclude a ligamentous injury.

KEY POINTS

■ The majority of injuries are shown on the *lateral film*

■ The following need to be checked:

  ▪ on the *lateral view*
    ❑ the top of T1 must be visible
    ❑ the three smooth arcs should be maintained
    ❑ the vertebral bodies are of uniform height
    ❑ the odontoid peg is intact and closely applied to C1

  ▪ on the *long AP view*
    ❑ the spinous processes are in a straight line and spaced equally apart

  ▪ on the *open mouth AP peg view*
    ❑ the base of the peg is intact
    ❑ the lateral margins of C1 and C2 align
    ❑ the spaces on either side of the peg are equal.

Remember

■ An important neck injury may still be present despite normal plain films. Clinical history and examination must always take precedence over apparently normal radiographs (ref. 10).

■ If the patient is otherwise well but there is severe pain and spasm and normal radiographs . . . book the patient for delayed views.

References

1. Hoffman JR, Schriger DL, Mower W, Luo JS, Zucker M. Low-risk criteria for cervical spine radiography in blunt trauma: a prospective study. *Ann Emerg Med* 1992, **21:** 1454–1460.
2. Roberge RJ, Wears RC, Kelly M, Evans TC, Kenny MA, Daffner R, Kremen R, Murray K, Cottington EC. Selective application of cervical spine radiography in alert victims of blunt trauma: a prospective study. *J Trauma* 1988, **28:** 784–788.
3. Doris PE, Wilson RA. The next logical step in the emergency radiographic evaluation of cervical spine trauma: the five view trauma series. *J. Emerg Med* 1985, **3:** 371–385.
4. Turetsky DB, Vines FS, Clayman DA, Northup HM. Technique and use of supine oblique views in acute cervical spine trauma. *Ann Emerg Med* 1993, **22:** 685–689.
5. Naidich JB, Naidich TP, Garfein C, Liebeskind AL, Hyman RA. The widened interspinous distance: a useful sign of anterior cervical dislocation in the supine frontal projection. *Radiology* 1977, **123:** 113–116.
6. Holliman CJ, Mayer JS, Cook RT, Smith JS. Is the anteroposterior cervical spine radiograph necessary in initial trauma screening? *Am J Emerg Med* 1991, **9:** 421–425.
7. Miles KA, Finlay D. Is prevertebral soft tissue swelling a useful sign in injury of the cervical spine? *Injury* 1988, **19:** 177–179.
8. Harris JH, Yeakley JS. Radiographically subtle soft tissue injuries of the cervical spine. *Current Problems in Diagnostic Radiology* 1989, **18:** 161–192.
9. Keats TE. *Atlas of Normal Roentgen Variants that may Simulate Disease*, 5th edition. Year Book Medical Publishers, Chicago, 1991.
10. Jones KE, Rawlinson JN. Managing neck injuries. *Br Med J* 1993, **307:** 868–869.
11. Daffner RH. Pseudofracture of the Dens: Mach bands. *Am J Roent* 1977, **128:** 607–612.

9 THORACIC AND LUMBAR SPINE

Severe disruption of the thoracic and lumbar spine invariably results from a very violent force. It will be clinically apparent that a serious injury has been sustained. It is not within the remit of this book to describe the full range of plain film appearances which may be found (Ref. 1) in these critically injured patients.

This short description is designed primarily to assist with the assessment of thoracic and lumbar spine radiographs in those patients who on clinical examination appear to have sustained a minor injury only.

BASIC RADIOGRAPHS

- Lateral.
- AP.

NORMAL ANATOMY

Lateral view

- The vertebral bodies are the same height, both anteriorly and posteriorly.
- The posterior margin of each vertebral body is slightly concave.

AP view

- In the thoracic region the paraspinal line (Figs 9.1 and 9.2) should be closely applied to the vertebral bodies.
- In the lumbar region the distance between the pedicles (Fig. 9.3) should become gradually wider from L1 to L5.

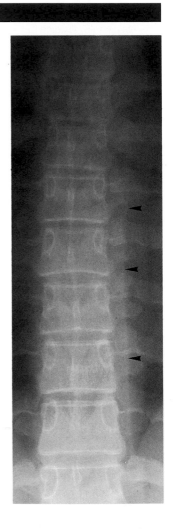

Figure 9.1. *The normal paraspinal line.*

Figure 9.2. *The normal paraspinal line (dark grey and arrows) is seen adjacent to the left lateral margin of the vertebral bodies. The light grey shadow situated more laterally is the normal descending aorta.*

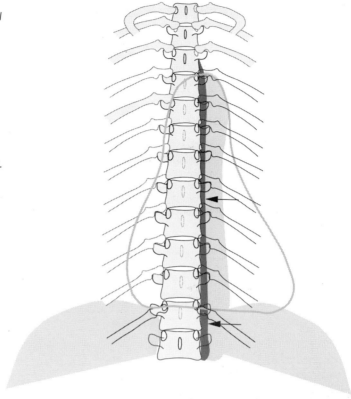

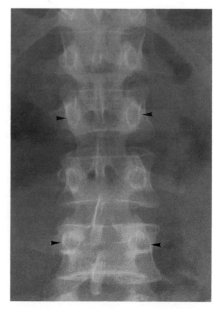

Figure 9.3. *The normal pedicles (arrowheads). The pedicles of L4 are normally slightly wider apart than those of L2.*

INJURIES

The clinical significance of an apparently simple wedge fracture may be underestimated. Occasionally the fracture is extensive with displacement of fragments into the spinal canal. Some of these patients may not demonstrate any neurological abnormality when first examined.

On the lateral view look for:

■ Loss of height or wedging of a vertebral body indicating a compression fracture (Fig. 9.4). This may be associated with loss of the normal concavity of the posterior aspect of the vertebral body; this finding indicates a significant posterior component to the fracture (Fig. 9.5).

■ Fragment(s) of bone detached from the anterior aspect of a vertebral body (Fig. 9.6).

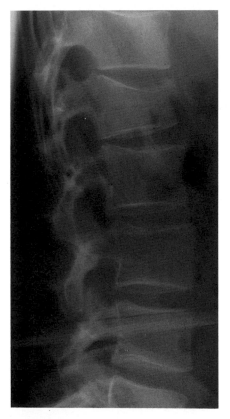

Figure 9.4 Wedge compression fracture of L1. The normal posterior concavity of the vertebral body is preserved.

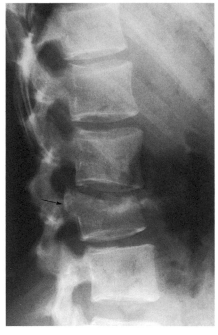

Figure 9.5. Wedge fracture of L3. The normal posterior concavity of the vertebral body is lost. Bone fragments (arrow) have been displaced into the spinal canal. This is an unstable fracture. (The patient had fallen from a horse three days previously, and had been able to continue at work despite back pain. There were no neurological signs.)

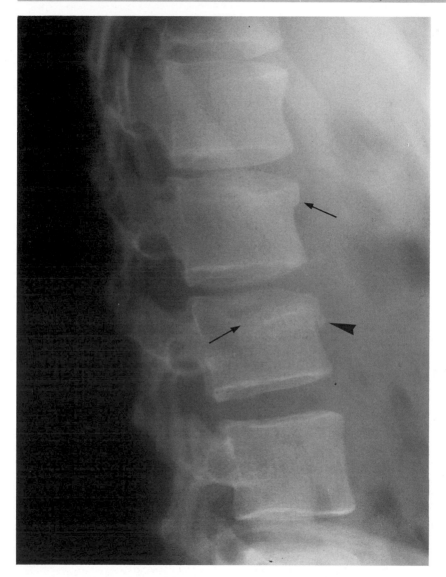

Figure 9.6. *Wedge compression fractures of L2 and L3 (arrows). A bone fragment has also been detached from the anterior aspect of L3 (arrowhead).*

On the AP view look for:

■ Displacement or widening of the paraspinal line in the thoracic region (Figs 9.7 and 9.8). In the context of trauma, this should be regarded as indicating a paraspinal haematoma resulting from a fracture.

■ Abnormal widening of the distance between the pedicles (Fig 9.9). This indicates that the fracture fragments have splayed apart.

■ Fractures of the transverse processes. These can be subtle injuries and often require the use of a bright light to assist detection.

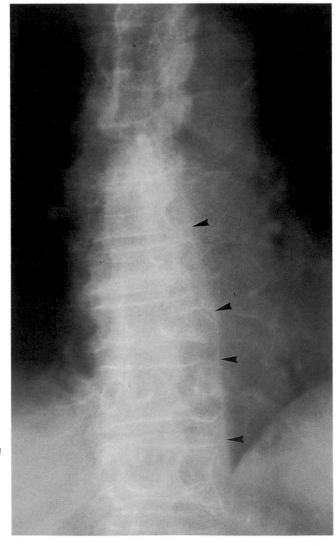

Figure 9.7. *Lateral bulge of the paraspinal line in the lower thoracic region due to a haematoma. This patient had sustained fractures of T9, T10 and T12 vertebrae.*

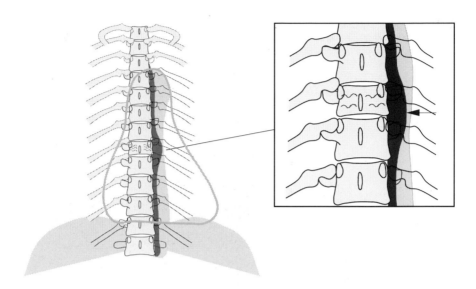

Figure 9.8. *The paraspinal line is displaced laterally in the mid-thoracic region. This is due to the haematoma around the T8 fracture.*

Figure 9.9. *Widening of the distance between the pedicles of L3 when compared with the interpediculate distance of the vertebral body below. This is the reverse of normal, and indicates a fracture. (This is the AP view of the patient shown in Fig 9.5.)*

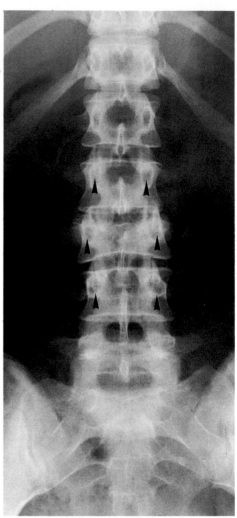

KEY POINTS

■ Most serious injuries result from an extremely violent force. The severity of injury is usually clinically obvious.

■ Very occasionally a serious injury may not be clinically obvious. **Check that:**

　▣ The vertebral bodies are of equal height.

　▣ The posterior margin of each vertebral body is slightly concave.

　▣ In the thoracic spine – the soft tissue paraspinal line does not bulge.

　▣ In the lumbar spine – the distance between the pedicles shows the normal slight widening when descending from L1 to L 5.

Reference

1. Pathria MN, Petersilge CA . Spinal trauma. *Radiol Clin North Am* 1991, **29:** 847–865.

10 PELVIS

BASIC RADIOGRAPHS

- AP view. This is one of the few sites where it is standard practice to obtain only one view.

IMPORTANT ANATOMY

- The pelvis (Fig. 10.1) comprises three bony rings:
    - The main pelvic ring.
    - Two smaller rings formed by the pubic and ischial bones.
- The sturdy sacro-iliac joints and the pubic symphysis are part of the main bony ring.
- The synchondrosis (i.e. the cartilaginous junction) between each ischial and pubic bone can sometimes appear confusing (Fig. 10.2). In early childhood these may simulate fracture lines. Between the ages of 5 and 7 years they may mimic healing fractures.

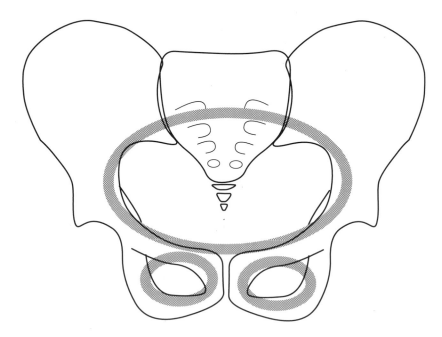

Figure 10.1. *The three pelvic rings.*

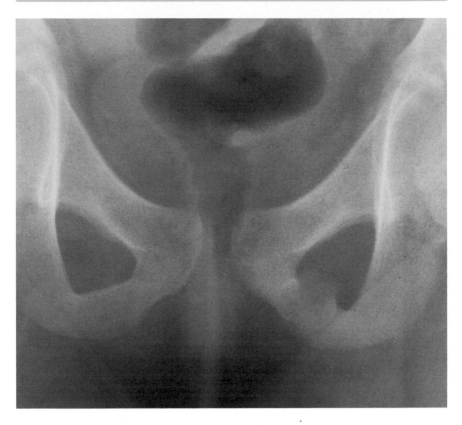

Figure 10.2. *Ossification of cartilage at the junction of the left ischial and pubic bones in a young child. This normal appearance can occur on one or both sides. It may be mistaken for a healing fracture.*

SYSTEMATIC INSPECTION OF THE AP FILM

'One fracture in a bony ring is frequently associated with a second fracture'.

Inspect the following:

- Main pelvic ring. Scrutinize both the inner and outer margins.
- The two secondary rings.
- Sacro-iliac joints. Compare their widths. These should be equal (Fig. 10.3).
- Symphysis pubis. The superior surfaces of the pubic rami should align (Fig. 10.3). The width of the joint should be approximately 5 mm.
- Sacral foramina (Figs 10.3 and 10.4). Disruption of any of these arcuate lines indicates a sacral fracture.
- The region of the acetabulum. This is a complex area and fractures are easy to overlook. Compare the appearance with that on the opposite uninjured side.

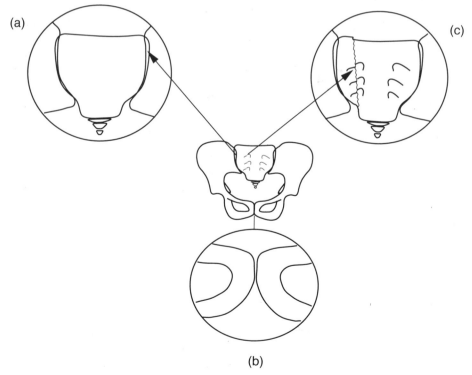

Figure 10.3. (a) *The width of the sacro-iliac joints should be equal.* **(b)** *The superior surfaces of the pubic rami should align.* **(c)** *The sacral foramina appear as curved white lines. Disruption of any of these curved sacral lines indicates a fracture. In this illustration there is a fracture of the right side of the sacrum.*

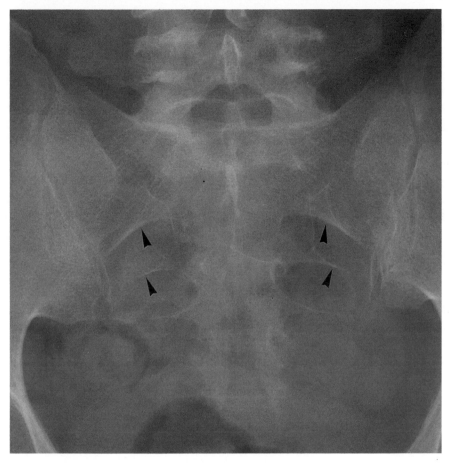

Figure 10.4. *The normal curved white lines forming the margins of the sacral foramina.*

Fractures involving a bony ring

■ A fracture at one point in a ring is likely to be associated with a second fracture elsewhere in the ring (Fig. 10.5).

■ A widened sacro-iliac joint, or a widened pubic symphysis, represents a fracture of the main ring (Fig. 10.6).

■ A double break in a ring should be regarded as an unstable injury.

■ Even though a fracture through a bone is not present, a combination of widening (diastasis) of the symphysis pubis and a sacro-iliac joint constitutes a double break in the main ring and therefore an unstable injury (Fig. 10.6).

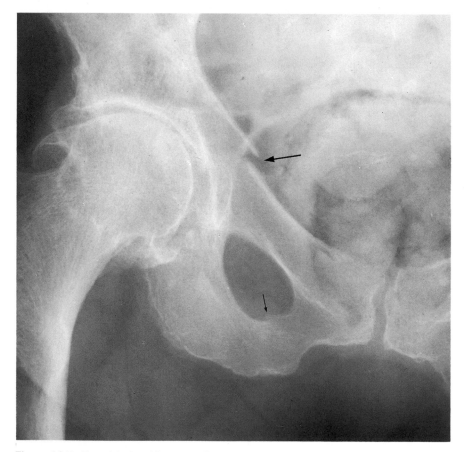

Figure 10.5. *Though isolated fractures of the smaller pubic rings do occur, it is common for a second fracture (small arrow) to be present.*

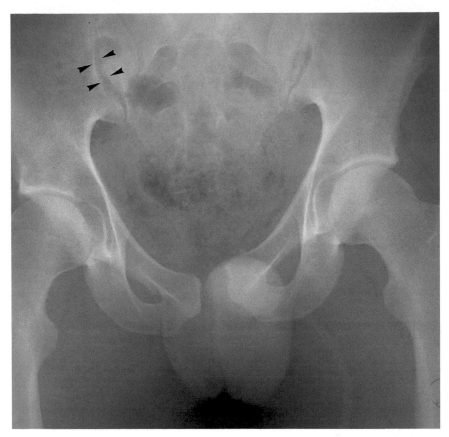

Figure 10.6. *Disruption of the symphysis pubis: the superior surfaces do not align and the joint is wider than 5 mm. In addition, the right sacro-iliac joint (arrowheads) is widened when compared with the uninjured opposite side.*

Other fractures

■ **Acetabular.** These (Fig. 10.7) are clinically important. If undetected, and subsequently improperly managed, they may result in premature degenerative change at the hip. This fracture is usually comminuted. Bone fragments may be trapped within the joint.

■ **Sacral.** These can be very difficult to detect. The arcuate lines (Figs 10.3 and 10.8) need to be carefully assessed, comparing one side with the other.

■ **Coccygeal.**

History: Fell on backside and the coccyx is tender.

In practice: The normal coccyx may appear very abnormal. In any case the radiographic findings do not affect management.

Advice: A radiograph is unnecessary.

■ **Avulsion.** These fractures (Figs 10.9 and 10.10) are most commonly caused by muscle contraction. They are usually the result of chronic stress in young athletes.

Common sites for avulsion fractures	Muscle origin
Anterior inferior iliac spine	Rectus femoris
Anterior superior iliac spine	Sartorius
Ischial tuberosity	Adductor magnus

Figure 10.7.
Fracture of the right ischium and fractures of the left superior and inferior pubic rami. These represent fractures of both the main pelvic ring as well as of the smaller ring. The abnormally wide symphysis pubis indicates that there is also a second break in the main ring, and this pelvis is unstable. It is easy to overlook the acetabular fracture (arrows).

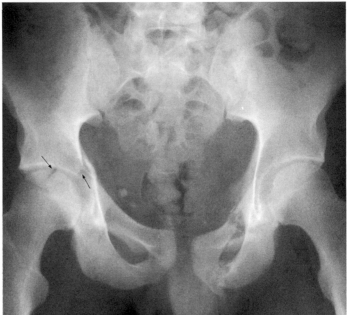

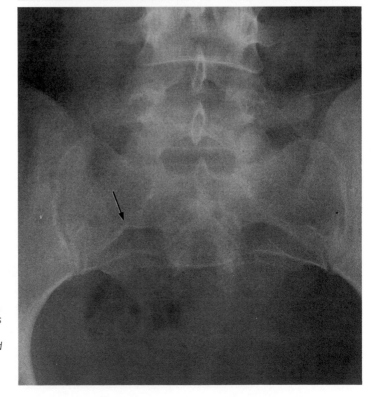

Figure 10.8.
Fracture through a sacral foramen. The white line is buckled (arrow) when compared with the other normal curved lines.

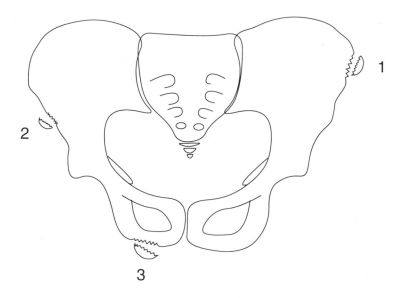

Figure 10.9. *In adolescence severe muscle contraction can detach a bone fragment from: (1) the anterior superior iliac spine, (2) the anterior inferior iliac spine, (3) the ischial tuberosity.*

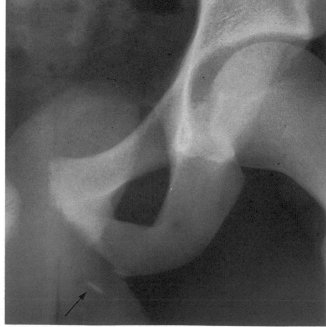

Figure 10.10. *An avulsion fracture of the ischial tuberosity.*

KEY POINTS

■ There are three bony rings. Bony rings frequently fracture at two sites.

■ Widening of a sacroiliac joint and/or the pubic symphysis may be the site of the second fracture.

■ Acetabular fractures are very important, but can be difficult to detect.

■ Sacral fractures are also difficult to detect . . . assess the arcuate lines.

■ Coccygeal fractures are very difficult to demonstrate . . . but radiographic confirmation is usually *unimportant*.

11 HIP AND PROXIMAL FEMUR

(For the paediatric hip see page 240)

BASIC RADIOGRAPHS

- AP of the whole pelvis including both hip joints.
- Lateral of the painful hip.

Points to note

- A fracture of a pubic ramus can mimic the symptoms and signs of a femoral neck fracture. The AP view of the whole pelvis allows assessment of the pubic rami on the two sides.

- A lateral view of the painful hip is essential. Some femoral neck fractures are impossible to detect on the AP view, but may be very obvious on the lateral view.

- Figure 11.1 shows how the femur is positioned during radiography, and explains why the lateral view (Fig. 11.2) can sometimes seem confusing.

- Underexposure (film too light) of the lateral radiograph is unacceptable. Inadequate films need to be repeated, otherwise fractures will be overlooked.

- Overexposure (film too dark) of the greater trochanter on the AP film of the pelvis is often unavoidable. When this occurs, the area must be examined with the aid of a bright light (Fig. 11.3).

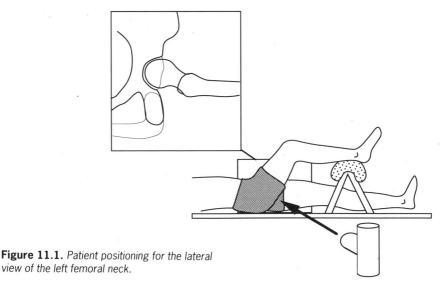

Figure 11.1. *Patient positioning for the lateral view of the left femoral neck.*

Figure 11.2. *Lateral view, normal.*

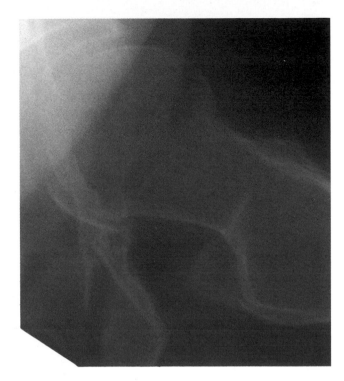

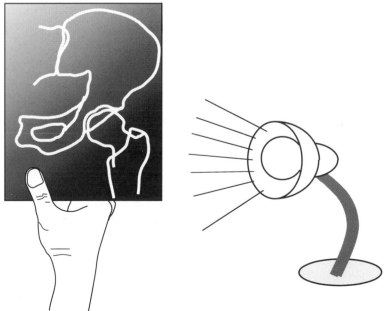

Figure 11.3. *A bright light is often necessary when assessing the greater trochanter.*

INJURIES

Fractures

■ Fractures of the femoral neck and proximal femur are common, and occur at characteristic sites (Fig. 11.4).

■ Most fractures are widely displaced and easy to detect.

■ **A few fractures are very difficult to detect.** If the radiographs appear superficially normal, it is important to answer the following questions:

    ▦ Are the cortices continuous or is there a slight step (Fig. 11.5)?

    ▦ Is the trabecular pattern continuous, or is it interrupted (Fig. 11.5)?

    ▦ Does a dense white line cross the femoral neck (Fig. 11.6)?

    ▦ Is there a fracture of a pubic ramus (Fig. 11.7)?

■ **Some undisplaced fractures may be totally undetectable on the initial radiograph.** Next steps: if there is a strong clinical suspicion of a fracture, and the x-ray findings are thought to be normal, then consider admitting the patient and repeating the radiograph two days later. Most fractures will be visible. If the radiograph is still normal but clinical suspicion remains high, an isotope bone scan will confirm or exclude a fracture.

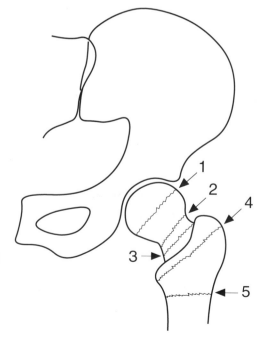

Figure 11.4. *Fractures of the proximal femur. The site of fracture affects both prognosis and management (ref. 1). Characteristic sites: subcapital 1, transcervical 2, basicervical 3, intertrochanteric 4, subtrochanteric 5.*

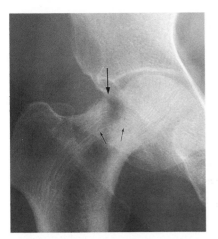 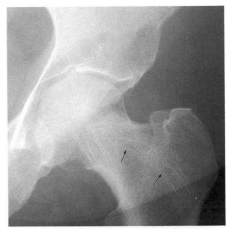

Figure 11.5. *The subcapital fracture (right) is identified by (a) the break in the cortical outline (large arrow) and (b) the interruption in the white lines which represent the trabeculae (small arrows). Compare these appearances with the normal trabeculae of the left femoral neck.*

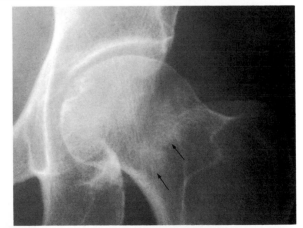

Figure 11.6. *Impacted fracture, identified by the sclerotic white line.*

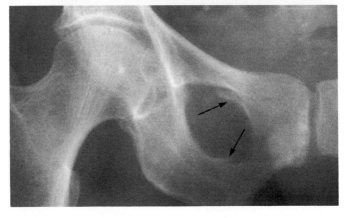

Figure 11.7. *Elderly patient fell and complained of pain in the right hip. The femoral neck is intact but there are fractures of the pubic rami.*

Dislocations

- These injuries follow very severe trauma and are unlikely to be overlooked.

- Dislocations can be posterior, anterior, or central. Most (80%) are posterior (Fig. 11.8). An associated fracture of the acetabulum is a common finding.

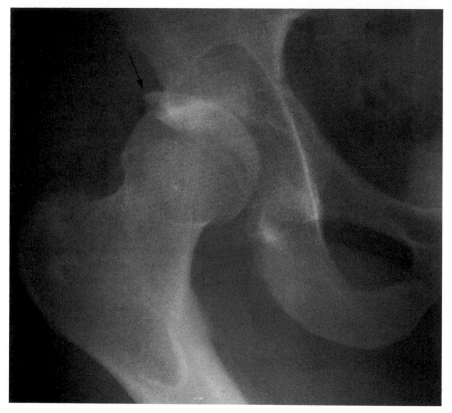

Figure 11.8. *Posterior dislocation of the head of the femur. Note the associated fracture of the acetabulum (arrow).*

KEY POINTS

■ An AP view of the whole pelvis is mandatory. Because:

  ▪ A fracture of a pubic ramus may mimic the pain of a femoral neck fracture.

  ▪ It allows comparison with the uninjured side.

■ A lateral view is also mandatory. A fracture involving the femoral neck and/or the trochanteric region may only be detectable on this view.

■ An impacted fracture may show as a dense white line only.

■ Slightly overexposed radiographs need to be scrutinized with a bright light.

Reference

1. Parker MJ, Pryor GA. *Hip Fracture Management*. Blackwell Scientific, Oxford, 1993.

12 KNEE

BASIC RADIOGRAPHS

- AP.
- lateral.

INJURIES

- Most patients who sustain a severe ligamentous or meniscal injury will have normal plain films.
- Most fractures are easy to detect.
- Occasionally, the only sign of an intra-articular fracture will be a fat fluid level in the suprapatellar bursa. The positioning of the injured patient (Fig. 12.1) explains why this sign only occurs on the lateral view
    - the lateral radiograph is usually obtained with the patient supine, utilizing a horizontal x-ray beam. This may show a knee joint effusion distending the suprapatellar bursa and displacing the patella away from the femur. This effusion may contain fat which has been released from the bone marrow by a fracture. The fat will lie on top of the underlying fluid (blood) resulting in a fat–fluid level.(Fig. 12.2).
    - a fat–fluid level within the suprapatellar bursa should be regarded as indicating an intra-articular fracture – even if a fracture is not seen.

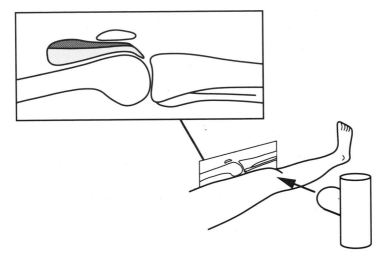

Figure 12.1. *The lateral view of the knee is usually obtained with a horizontal x-ray beam. In this patient a fat–fluid level is present. Fat (dark shading) lies on top of blood (light shading) in the suprapatellar bursa.*

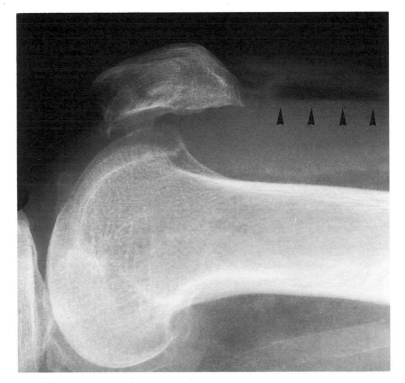

Figure 12.2. *Lipohaemarthrosis. Bone marrow fat has entered the suprapatellar bursa from an intra-articular fracture.*

Fractures – tibial plateau

■ These fractures (Fig. 12.3) are often associated with significant damage to either the medial collateral ligament and/or the cruciate ligaments.

■ Eighty percent are seen as a depression in the lateral tibial plateau due to forced impaction by the lateral femoral condyle. The so-called car bumper injury. A similar injury to the medial plateau does occur but is less common.

■ **Important clue:** in some cases an impacted fracture of the tibial plateau may only be visible as an area of increased bone density (Figs 12.4 and 12.5). Oblique views may be very useful, indeed essential, to confirm the diagnosis.

■ **Useful clue:** on the AP view of the normal knee the femoral condyles and upper tibia align (Fig. 12.6). In the presence of a plateau fracture the tibial margin is often displaced so that there is a step at the level of the knee joint (Figs 12.5–12.7). The following rule can be applied: a perpendicular line drawn at the most lateral margin of the femur should not have more than five millimetres of the adjacent margin of the tibia beyond it. If this rule is broken then a fracture of the lateral tibial plateau should be suspected (Fig. 12.6).

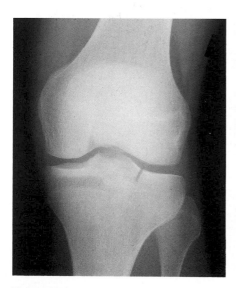

Figure 12.3. *Fracture through the lateral tibial plateau.*

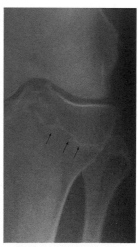

Figure 12.4. *Tibial plateau fracture. The dense white area (arrows) is subtle – but it is evidence of a compression fracture of the lateral condyle of the tibia.*

Figure 12.5. *Fracture through the lateral tibial plateau. Though there is disruption of the articular surface of the tibia, the fracture is also indicated because of* **(a)** *the increased density of the impacted bone, and* **(b)** *the malalignment (arrows) resulting from the lateral displacement of the lateral tibial condyle (see Fig. 12.6.)*

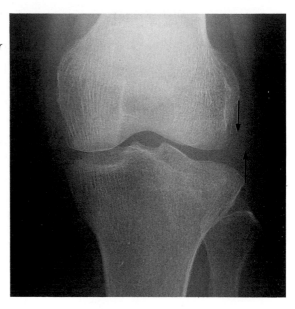

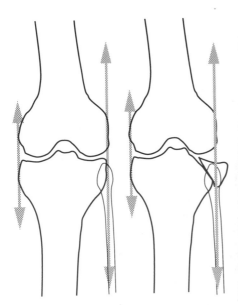

Figure 12.6. *In the normal knee (left) a perpendicular line drawn at the most lateral margin of the femur should have no more than 5 mm of adjacent tibia outside of it. When this rule is broken a plateau fracture (right) is a possibility.*

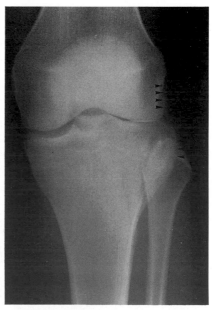

Figure 12.7. *Tibial plateau fracture. The fracture line is partially obscured by the head of the fibula. Note: the lateral femoral condyle does not align normally with the lateral tibial margin (arrowheads).*

Fractures – patella

- A direct blow is the usual cause of a comminuted fracture (Fig. 12.8).

- Severe muscle spasm can cause a transverse fracture (Fig. 12.9).

- Some fractures will not be shown on either of the standard views of the knee. If a fracture of the patella is strongly suspected on clinical examination, and the AP and lateral views appear normal, then a further view is necessary, either a skyline view (Fig. 12.10) or an oblique view (ref. 1).

- An unfused secondary ossification centre – a bipartite patella – may mimic a fracture (Fig. 12.11).

- A bipartite patella:

    - is characteristically situated in the upper outer quadrant;

    - has well-defined margins.

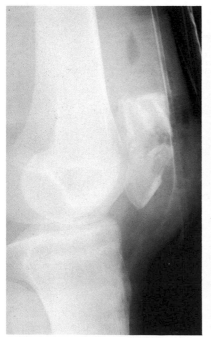

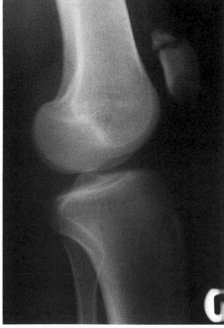

Figure 12.8. *Comminuted fracture of the patella.*

Figure 12.9. *Transverse fracture of the patella.*

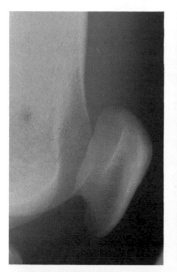
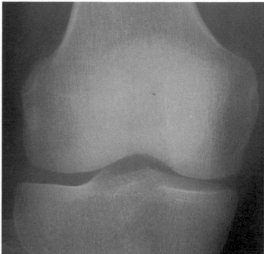
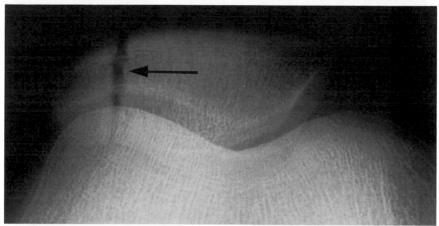

Figure 12.10. *Some patellar fractures (arrow) are impossible to identify on the standard AP and lateral views. If there is clinical suspicion of a patellar injury and the two standard radiographs appear normal then an additional view of the patella should be obtained.*

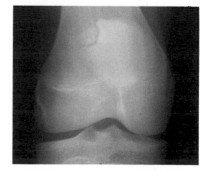

Figure 12.11. *Bipartite patella. This is a normal variant and should not be confused with a fracture. The margins are sclerotic and well defined. The position in the upper outer quadrant is characteristic.*

Fractures – fibular neck

An *Isolated* fracture of the head, or neck, of the fibula is uncommon (Fig. 12.12). This fracture is commonly associated with another knee injury – either damage to the collateral or cruciate ligaments, or another fracture around the knee joint (Fig. 12.13).

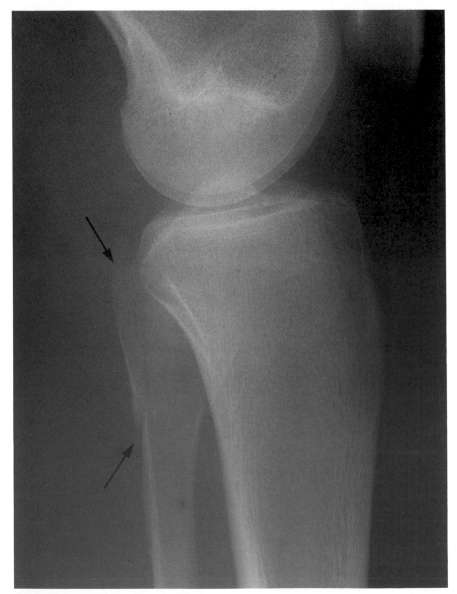

Figure 12.12. *An isolated fracture of the neck of the fibula.*

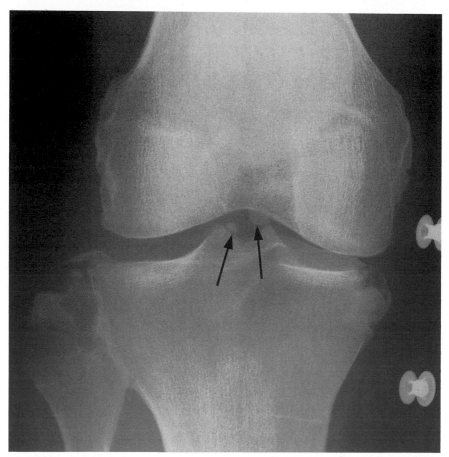

Figure 12.13. *A fracture involving the neck of the fibula is often associated with other injuries to the knee joint. There are multiple fractures present in this patient.*

Fractures – associated with a cruciate ligament injury

The cruciate ligaments insert into the intercondylar region of the tibial plateau. Ligamentous rupture does not usually include a fracture. Occasionally the bony insertions may be avulsed, and bone fragments may then become visible within the joint (Figs 12.13 and 12.14).

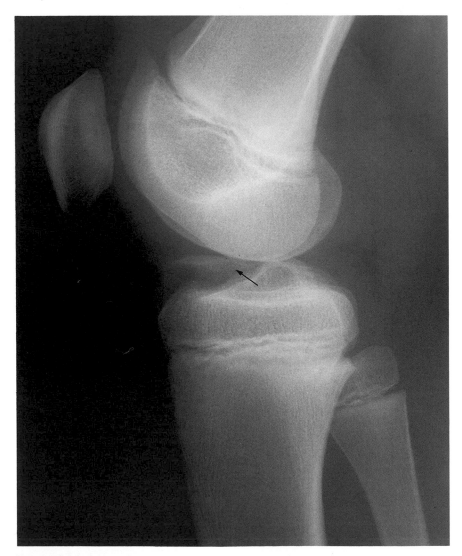

Figure 12.14. *Avulsion fracture at the insertion of the anterior cruciate ligament.*

KEY POINTS

■ Most fractures are obvious.

■ A normal radiograph does not exclude a severe ligamentous or cartilaginous injury.

■ If the lateral film shows a fat-fluid level in the suprapatellar bursa then this indicates an intra-articular fracture.

■ Tibial plateau fractures can be subtle. Look for:

  ▪ an area of increased bone density;

  ▪ displacement of the margin of the tibia.

■ Patellar fractures can be subtle. Oblique or skyline views may be required if the AP and lateral films appear normal.

■ Intra-articular bone fragments may indicate a severe injury, for example avulsion at the insertion of a cruciate ligament.

Reference

1. Daffner R H, Tabas J H. Trauma oblique radiographs of the knee. *J Bone Joint Surg* 1987, **69:** 568–571.

13 ANKLE AND HINDFOOT

The ankle is a ring structure of three bones (tibia, talus and fibula) linked by three ligaments (the medial and lateral collateral ligaments and the interosseous ligament). A break in one part of the ring is likely to result in a second break elsewhere.

The second break may be either another fracture or ligamentous damage.

BASIC RADIOGRAPHS

- **AP mortice:** obtained with slight internal rotation so that the fibula does not overlap the talus. This enables the lateral aspect of the joint space to be visualized (Fig 13.1).

- **Lateral:** to include the entire calcaneum and ideally the base of the fifth metatarsal (Fig. 13.2).

AP mortice view

Inspect:

- The joint space. It should be traced from the medial side, over the superior aspect of the talus, to the lateral side of the joint. This space should be uniform all the way around (Fig. 13.1).

- The integrity of the talar dome.

Lateral view

Inspect:

- The lateral and medial malleoli (Fig. 13.2). The lateral malleolus extends more inferiorly than does the medial malleolus.

- The posterior aspect of the tibia – sometimes termed the posterior malleolus.

- The calcaneum. A calcaneal fracture may occasionally result from an apparently simple twisting injury.

- The fifth metatarsal. It is common for an inversion injury to cause an avulsion fracture at the base of this metatarsal.

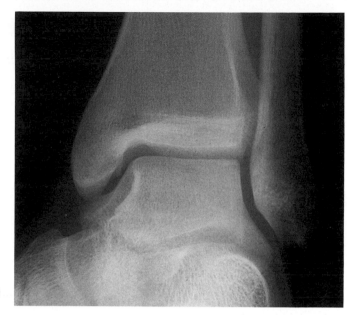

Figure 13.1.
Normal AP mortice view.

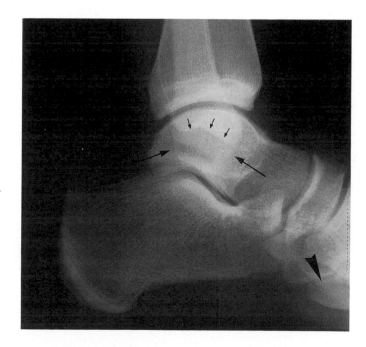

Figure 13.2.
Normal lateral view. The lateral malleolus (large arrows) is projected inferior to the medial malleolus (small arrows). Note that the entire calcaneum and the base of the fifth metatarsal (arrowhead) are included on the radiograph.

INJURIES

Ligamentous injuries around the mortice joint

■ The radiographs may appear normal even with severe ligamentous damage.

■ If there is widening of one side of the joint space (Fig. 13.3) then there is commonly an associated fracture elsewhere.

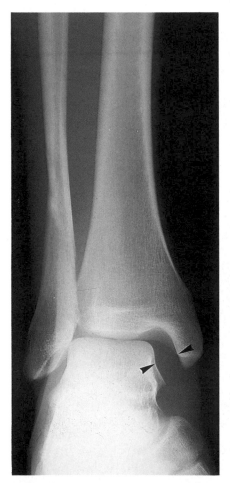 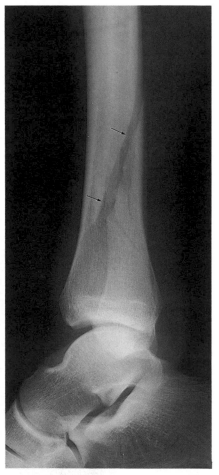

Figure 13.3. *The AP mortice view shows widening of the medial joint space (arrowheads) indicating damage to the medial collateral ligament. Since the bony/ligamentous ring has been ruptured at one position then a second injury should be sought. The lateral view shows an oblique fracture of the fibula (arrows).*

Fractures around the mortice joint

■ Are usually obvious. But:

  ▤ it is common for a fracture to be identified on one view only (Figs 13.3 and 13.4). The lateral view must be scrutinized very carefully – particularly for oblique fractures of the fibula, and for fractures involving the posterior aspect of the tibia (Fig. 13.4).

  ▤ if one fracture is seen, then it is important to look carefully for a second fracture, or joint space widening. The latter indicates ligamentous damage.

■ An osteochondral fracture of the talar dome may be identified by either a small bone fragment within the joint, or as a defect in the cortex of the talus (Fig. 13.5).

■ Epiphyseal plate (Salter–Harris) fractures are common. (See page 232).

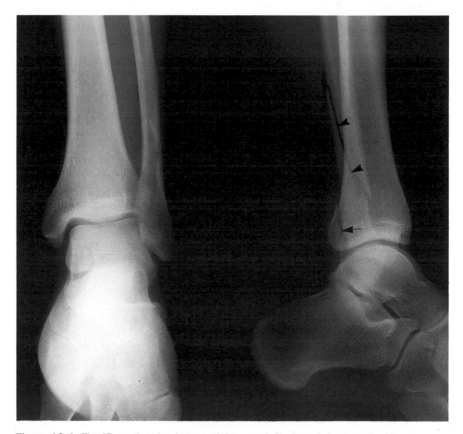

Figure 13.4. *The AP mortice view is essentially normal. The lateral view reveals oblique fractures of the fibula and of the posterior aspect of the tibia.*

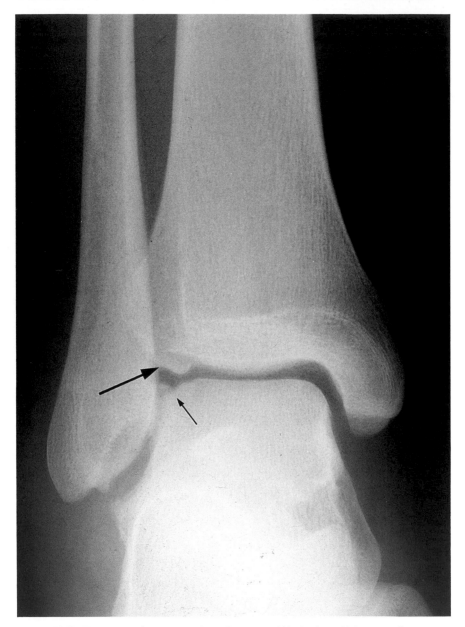

Figure 13.5. *The mortice view shows a bone fragment within the lateral joint space (large arrow). The cortex of the talar dome has lost its normal well-defined smooth contour (small arrow). These findings indicate an osteochondral fracture of the talus.*

Calcaneal fractures

■ Calcaneal fractures may result from an apparently simple twisting injury and not solely from a fall from a height.

■ All patients presenting with a history of a twisted ankle require careful clinical examination of the calcaneum.

■ If a calcaneal fracture is clinically suspected then an axial view should be obtained (Figs 13.6 and 13.7).

■ Radiographic appearances of calcaneal fractures:

  ▨ Most will be obvious on the lateral view.

  ▨ Some will only become apparent when Bohler's angle is assessed (Fig. 13.8). This angle normally measures 30–40 degrees. If a calcaneal fracture results in flattening of the bone then the angle will be reduced below 30 degrees (Figs 13.9 and 13.10).

  ▨ A normal Bohler's angle does not exclude a fracture.

  ▨ A sclerotic line in the calcaneum may represent an impacted fracture (Fig. 13.11).

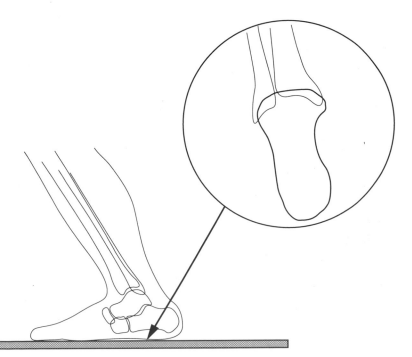

Figure 13.6. *Positioning of the patient for an axial view of the calcaneum.*

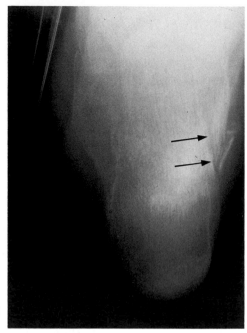

Figure 13.7. *Axial view of the calcaneum showing a fracture.*

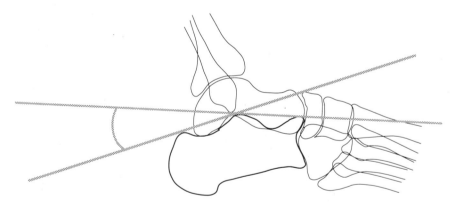

Figure 13.8. *Bohler's angle. This is assessed on the lateral ankle radiograph. It is measured by drawing a line from the posterior aspect of the calcaneum to its highest midpoint. A second line is drawn from this point to the highest anterior point. The angle to be measured is shown. Normal = 30–40 degrees.*

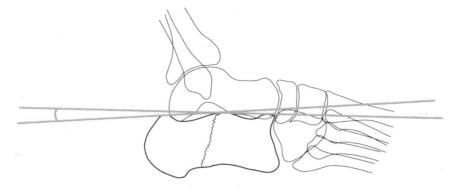

Figure 13.9. *Calcaneal fracture with compression. Bohler's angle is flattened.*

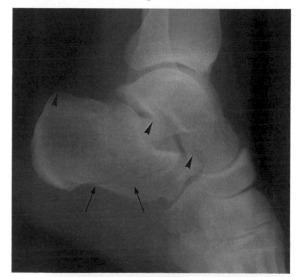

Figure 13.10. *The arrowheads indicate the points to be used when measuring Bohler's angle. Note that the angle is reduced. Part of the fracture is shown (arrows).*

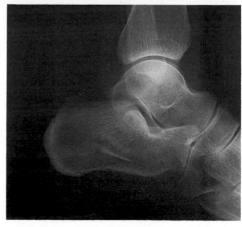

Figure 13.11. *Twisted ankle. The sclerotic (dense) line in the body of the calcaneum represents an impacted fracture. Note that Bohler's angle is normal.*

POTENTIAL PITFALLS

Accessory ossicles

■ Accessory ossicles (Fig. 13.12) adjacent to the tips of the medial and lateral malleoli are very common – as are fracture fragments. Sometimes it can be difficult to distinguish between them. Clinical correlation is important. Fractures are tender, accessory ossicles are not.

In addition:

▨ an accessory ossicle has a well defined (i.e. sclerotic) outline;

▨ a fracture fragment is usually ill defined on one of its sides.

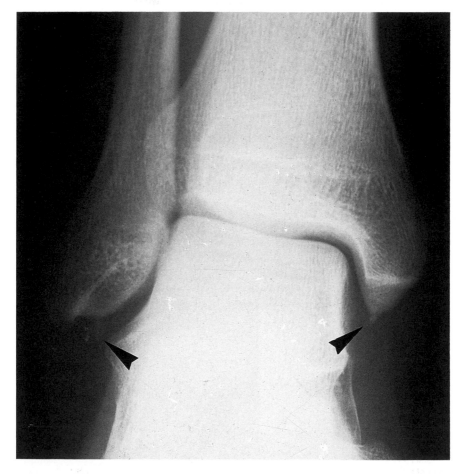

Figure 13.12. *The small bone fragments adjacent to the tip of the lateral and medial malleoli have well corticated outlines. These are unfused secondary centres and are common normal variants.*

Fracture of the base of the fifth metatarsal

■ A twisting injury of the ankle may result in an injury remote from the ankle joint. This should be remembered when examining the patient clinically and when inspecting the radiographs.

■ This is a common injury in patients presenting with a twisted ankle. It results from avulsion at the insertion of the peroneus brevis tendon (Fig. 13.13). The fracture (Fig. 13.14) occurs as a consequence of forced inversion.

■ Though this fracture is relatively common, routine ankle and foot radiography is discouraged. Careful clinical examination of the base of the fifth metatarsal will indicate when radiographs of the foot should be obtained instead of ankle views.

■ *In young patients the normal unfused apophysis at the base of the fifth metatarsal should not be misinterpreted as a fracture*

  ▓ a fracture line is usually transverse to the long axis of the metatarsal (Figs 13.13 and 13.14)

  ▓ an apophysis lies longitudinal to the long axis of the metatarsal (Figs 13.15 and 13.16).

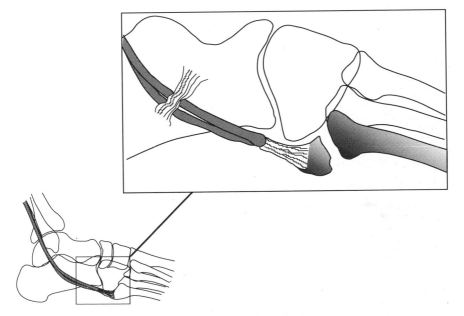

Figure 13.13. *Inversion injury. The peroneus brevis tendon inserts into the base of the fifth metatarsal. An avulsion fracture is shown.*

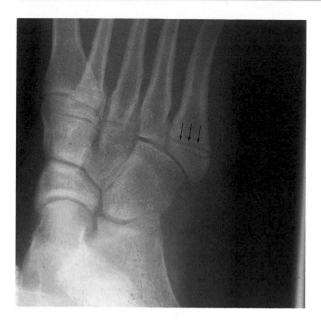

Figure 13.14.
Fracture of the base of the fifth metatarsal. Note that the fracture line runs at right angles to the cortex of the bone. This distinguishes it from a normal unfused apophysis. The long axis of the latter is parallel to the metatarsal.

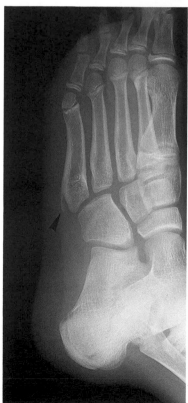

Figure 13.15. *Typical appearance of an unfused apophysis at the base of the fifth metatarsal.*

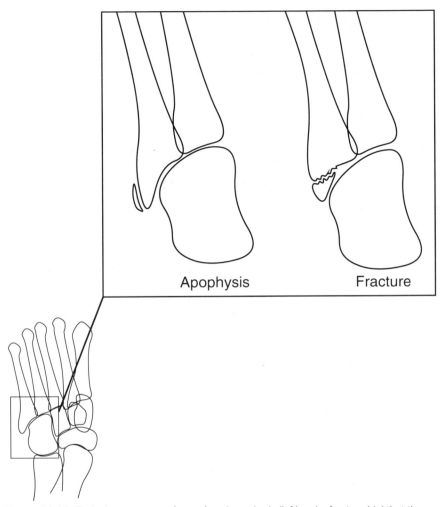

Figure 13.16. Typical appearance of an unfused apophysis (left) and a fracture (right) at the base of the fifth metatarsal.

Maissoneuve fracture

■ The ankle joint is a bony ring. Sometimes this ring extends to the knee.

■ An external rotation injury of the ankle may result in a high fracture of the *proximal shaft* of the fibula. The fibular fracture may be overlooked because the main symptoms are around the ankle joint (Fig. 13.17). This combination of injuries is known as a Maissoneuve fracture.

■ A Maissoneuve fracture should be suspected when there is *a seemingly isolated* fracture of the medial malleolus – or of the posterior malleolus – *accompanied by widening of the ankle joint space.*

■ Clinical examination of the upper leg is important in all patients attending with an ankle injury.

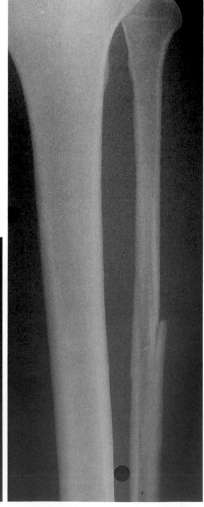

Figure 13.17. *Maissoneuve fracture. There is a fracture with subluxation at the ankle joint, and this is associated with a fracture of the proximal fibula.*

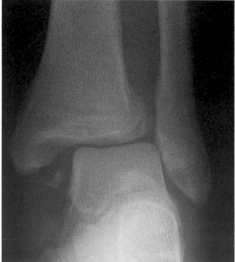

KEY POINTS

- Careful clinical examination of the entire hindfoot and upper leg is essential. A twisted ankle may result in a fracture of:
  - the base of the fifth metatarsal
  - the calcaneum
  - the upper fibula.
- An avulsion fracture at the base of the fifth metatarsal is common. This should not be confused with a normal unfused apophysyis.

    fracture – transverse to the long axis of the metatarsal

    apophysis – longitudinal to the long axis of the metatarsal.

- An osteochondral fracture of the dome of the talus is easy to overlook.

- Apply the guideline: *no need for routine foot films when the ankle alone is injured.*

14 MIDFOOT AND FOREFOOT

Many patients who have sustained a fracture of a metatarsal or a phalanx do not require radiography. Appropriate management can be determined from clinical examination alone. The x-ray findings whether positive or negative rarely influence management. Thus patients with an injury to the midfoot or forefoot who do not have gross signs or symptoms can be offered symptomatic treatment without the need for radiography (ref. 1).

BASIC RADIOGRAPHS

■ AP.

■ Oblique.

IMPORTANT ANATOMY

■ Several tarsal bones and the bases of the metatarsals overlap on the AP view. The oblique view produces some separation of these bones.

■ **Important rules:**

  ▪ The medial margin of the base of the **second** metatarsal should be in line with the medial margin of the middle cuneiform on the **AP view**.

  ▪ The medial margin of the base of the **third** metatarsal should be in line with the medial margin of the lateral cuneiform on the **oblique view**.

■ There are numerous accessory ossicles, but they rarely cause problems with interpretation (Fig. 14.1). Those appearances which may occasionally mimic a fracture are illustrated in *Keats' Atlas* (ref. 2).

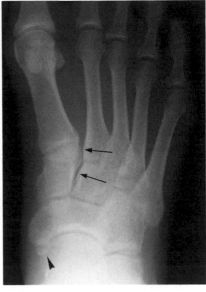

Figure 14.1. *AP view. Note: the medial margin of the second metatarsal (2) is in line with the medial margin of the middle cuneiform (arrows). The arrowhead points to a very common accessory ossicle (os tibiale externum).*

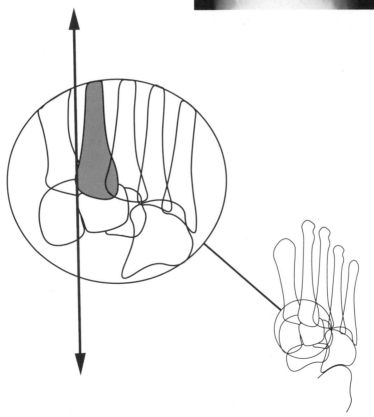

Figure 14.2. *Normal alignment at the tarso-metatarsal joints on the AP view.*

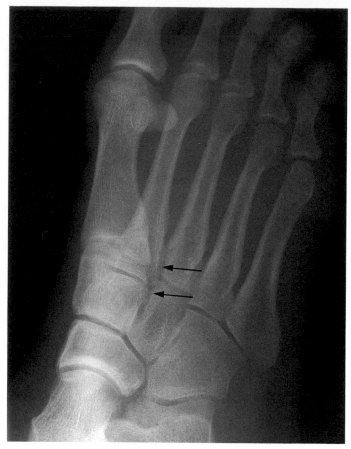

Figure 14.3. *Oblique view. Note: the medial margin of the third metatarsal (3) is in line with the medial margin of the lateral cuneiform (arrows). The base of the second metatarsal is obscured by overlapping bones.*

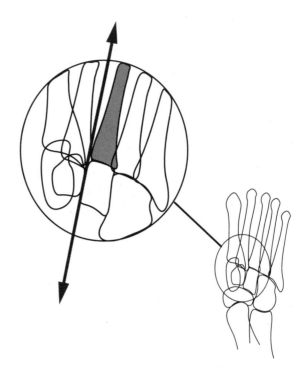

Figure 14.4. *Normal alignment at the tarso-metatarsal joints on the oblique view.*

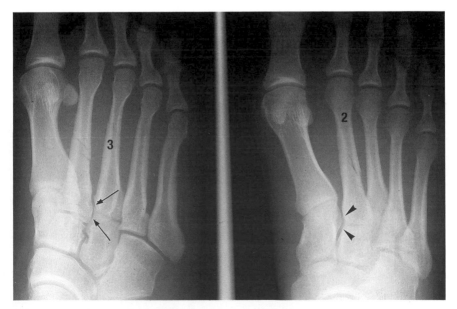

Figure 14.5. *Fracture through the shaft of the second metatarsal. Note the normal alignments at the Lisfranc (tarso-metatarsal) joints on the oblique (left) and AP (right) views.*

INJURIES

The midfoot

Tarsal fractures and dislocations

These are uncommon, and result from severe trauma. There will be little clinical doubt that there is a severe injury. It is usually easy to detect the important fractures and dislocations.

Tarso-metatarsal dislocations

■ These are easy to overlook.

■ Traumatic subluxations and dislocations at the bases of the metatarsals (Lisfranc injuries) will be difficult to detect if the observer is unfamiliar with the normal alignment of the bones.

■ If a bony fragment is detached from the base of any of the four medial metatarsals then a tarso-metatarsal dislocation (Fig. 14.6) should be suspected.

■ Minor tarso-metatarsal subluxations can be very difficult to identify (Fig. 14.7), and the AP and oblique views should always be inspected to confirm that the bony alignments are normal. There are two questions to answer:

■ On the AP view does the medial margin of the base of the second metatarsal align with the medial margin of the middle cuneiform?

■ On the oblique view does the medial margin of the third metatarsal align with the medial margin of the lateral cuneiform?'

■ Occasionally a fracture will occur through the second metatarsal distal to its base, but the base is held in place by the ligaments. The distal metatarsal fragment then dislocates laterally with the third, fourth and fifth metatarsals. *In this circumstance it is the alignment of the medial margin of the third metatarsal with the medial margin of the lateral cuneiform which is disrupted (Fig. 14.8).*

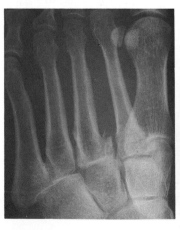
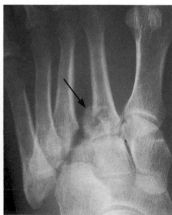

Figure 14.6. *Lisfranc injury. Metatarsal fracture (arrow). Note the loss of the normal alignment of the medial aspect of the base of the third metatarsal on the oblique view. The third, fourth and fifth metatarsals have subluxed laterally.*

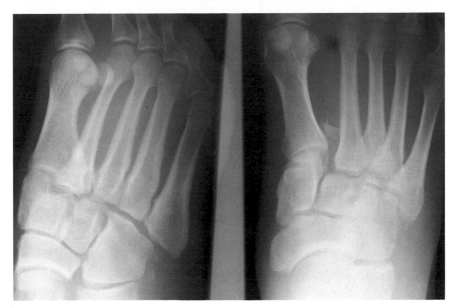

`Figure 14.7.` Lisfranc injury. There is loss of the
normal metatarsal–cuneiform alignments on both
the oblique (left) and AP (right) views.

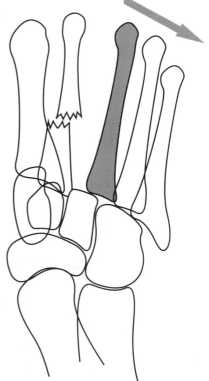

Figure 14.8. Lisfranc injury. A fracture through the
base of the second metatarsal with dislocation of
the third, fourth and fifth metatarsals shown on the
oblique view.

Potential pitfall: The second metatarsal base will
have maintained its normal alignment with the
middle cuneiform on the AP view.

The forefoot

Fracture of the base of the fifth metatarsal (See also page 169)

Recap:

■ A fracture of the base of the fifth metatarsal usually results from an inversion injury of the ankle.

■ Careful clinical examination of the base of the fifth metatarsal will indicate that foot, not ankle, radiographs should be requested.

■ **The normal unfused apophysis at the base of the fifth metatarsal should not be misinterpreted as a fracture.**

Stress fracture of a metatarsal

■ It is common for most but not all of these injuries to show some periosteal new bone formation (Fig. 14.9).

■ If clinical suspicion of a stress fracture is high and the initial radiographs appear normal, then it is worth considering requesting an isotope bone scan – but only if the result would affect patient management.

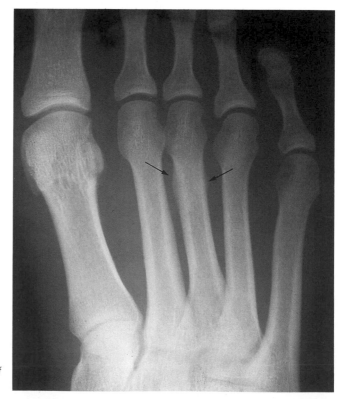

Figure 14.9. *Stress fracture. There is a periosteal reaction along the mid-shaft of the third metatarsal.*

KEY POINTS

Midfoot

■ Lisfranc midfoot subluxations or dislocations may be subtle, particularly in the absence of a fracture. *Check that the anatomy is normal:*

 ▨ *The medial margin of the base of the second metatarsal should line up with the medial margin of the middle cuneiform on the AP view.*

 ▨ *The medial margin of the base of the third metatarsal should line up with the medial margin of the lateral cuneiform on the oblique view.*

Forefoot

■ An avulsion fracture of the base of the fifth metatarsal is common and usually results from inversion of the ankle.

■ Consider the diagnosis of a metatarsal stress fracture even in the absence of obvious trauma.

References

1. David HG. Value of radiographs in managing common foot injuries. *Br Med J* 1989, **298:** 1491–1492.
2. Keats TE. *Atlas of Normal Roentgen Variants That May Simulate Disease*, 5th edition. Year Book Medical Publishers, Chicago, 1991.

15 CHEST

Chest radiography is very important in accident and emergency medicine. A comprehensive description of the radiology of thoracic emergencies belongs in a much larger textbook (ref. 1). In the space available here it is not possible even to summarise the many medical and surgical emergencies that may be encountered. Therefore we have deliberately limited our description to three of the more common clinical problems.

RIB FRACTURES

- Assuming that the clinical examination suggests a relatively minor injury to the thorax:
  - A chest radiograph is obtained solely to exclude an important complication such as a pneumothorax.
  - Oblique views of the ribs are not necessary because clinical management is rarely altered by the demonstration of a fracture.

PNEUMOTHORAX

- An erect radiograph taken in full expiration is recommended. An expiration film usually enables a small pneumothorax to be identified most easily.
- The features to look for:
  - a clearly defined line which represents the edge of the lung. The line parallels the chest wall (Fig. 15.1).
  - the upper part of this line will be curved at the lung apex.
  - absence of lung markings (i.e. vessels) between the lung edge and the chest wall (Fig. 15.1).

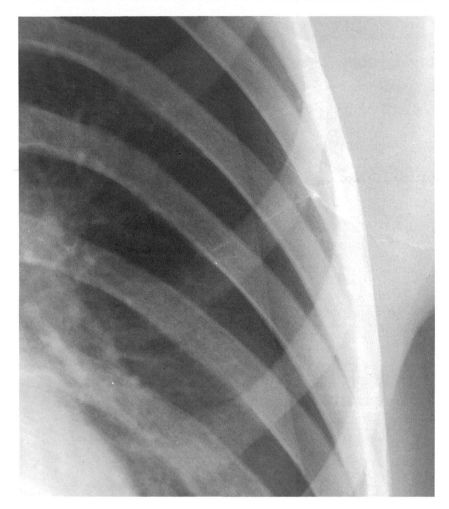

Figure 15.1. *Left-sided pneumothorax. Two features to note: there is a well-defined line which represents the lung edge, and there are no lung vessels lateral to this line.*

PNEUMONIA

Radiography

- If the patient's condition permits:
  - PA. Erect, in full inspiration.
  - A lateral view is occasionally obtained when seeking to clarify an abnormality seen on the PA film.
- Severely ill patient:
  - AP. Sitting semi-erect or lying supine.

Anatomy

- On the well-penetrated erect PA film (Fig. 15.2):
  - The left and right heart borders are well defined.
  - Both hemidiaphragms are visible almost to the midline.
- On the AP supine film:
  - A full inspiration is not always possible. A poor inspiration may result in:
    - ❏ apparent cardiac enlargement (Fig. 15.3);
    - ❏ increased basal shadows which can mimic inflammatory change (Fig. 15.4).
- On the lateral film (Fig. 15.5):
  - Both hemidiaphragms are visible posterior to the cardiac shadow.
  - The area behind the heart is approximately as black as the area behind the sternum.
  - The lower vertebral bodies appear darker compared with the vertebrae in the mid and upper thorax.
  - *If any of these rules are broken then lower lobe pathology, usually lung consolidation or a pleural effusion, is likely.*

Lung consolidation

A patient presenting with malaise, cough, or fever and few other clinical signs or symptoms is a common problem. Pneumonia needs to be excluded. Sometimes the radiographic features of consolidation are subtle (Fig. 15.6), and the chest film may appear normal. It is important to assess the mediastinal and diaphragmatic boundaries, and this can be done by answering the question:

> *'Are both heart borders and both hemidiaphragms well defined and clearly visible?'*

■ **If any of these borders are ill defined then pathology in the adjacent lung is likely.**

■ The site of consolidation in the lung can be deduced as shown in Table 15.1.

Table 15.1. Clues to the site of consolidation.

Ill defined:	Suspected site of consolidation:
Right heart border (Fig. 15.7)	Middle lobe
Left heart border (Figs 15.8 and 15.9)	Left upper lobe
Right hemidiaphragm (Fig. 15.10)	Right lower lobe
Left hemidiaphragm (Figs 15.6 and 15.11)	Left lower lobe

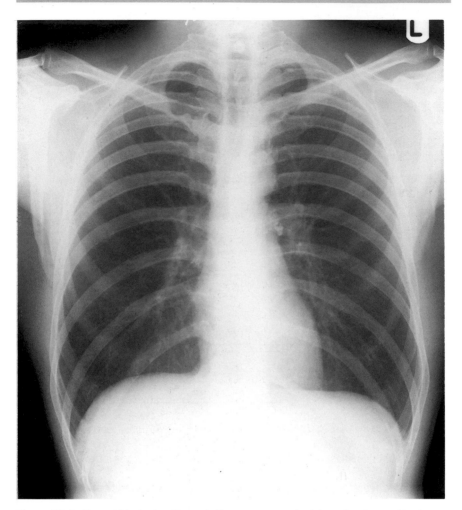

Figure 15.2. *Normal PA chest radiograph. Features to note: both heart borders and both hemidiaphragms are sharp and well defined.*

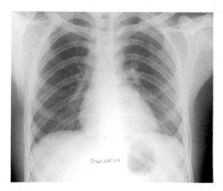
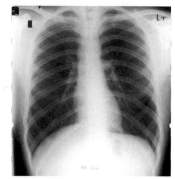

Figure15.3. *Effect of a poor inspiration. The transverse cardiac diameter exceeds 50% of the diameter of the chest (left) and raises the possibility of cardiac enlargement. The film was repeated a few minutes later (right) following a full inspiration. The transverse cardiac diameter is now normal.*

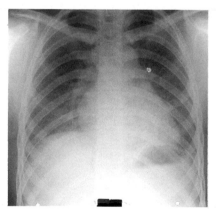
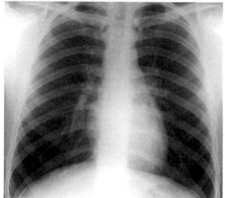

Figure 15.4. *Effect of a poor inspiration. Increased basal shadowing suggests lower zone consolidation (left). Repeat film five minutes later (right) following a full inspiration. The lungs are clear.*

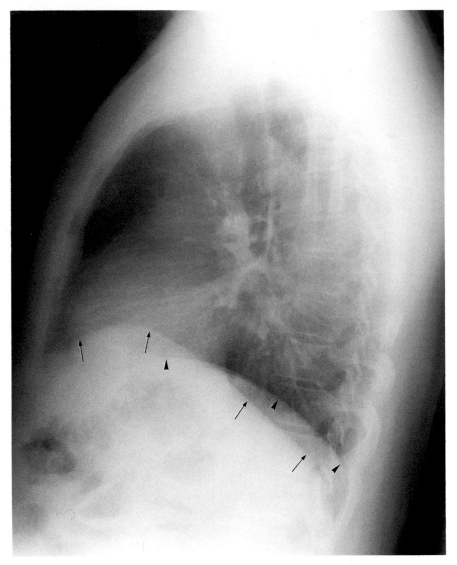

Figure 15.5. *Normal lateral radiograph. Features to note: (1) both hemidiaphragms are seen (right dome = arrows, left dome = arrowheads) (2) the density (film blackening) behind the heart and behind the sternum are approximately equal, (3) the lower thoracic vertebral bodies appear darker than those in the mid- and upper-thorax.*

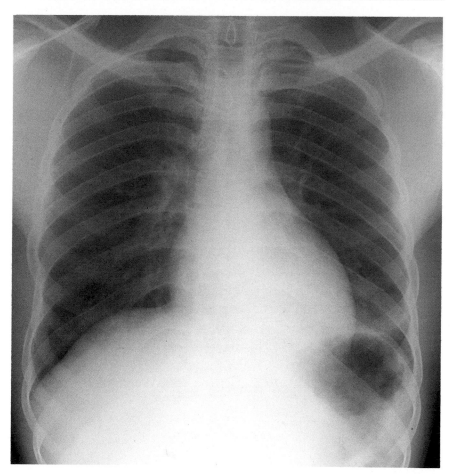

Figure 15.6. *Left lower lobe consolidation. The medial aspect of the left hemidiaphragm is not sharply defined.*

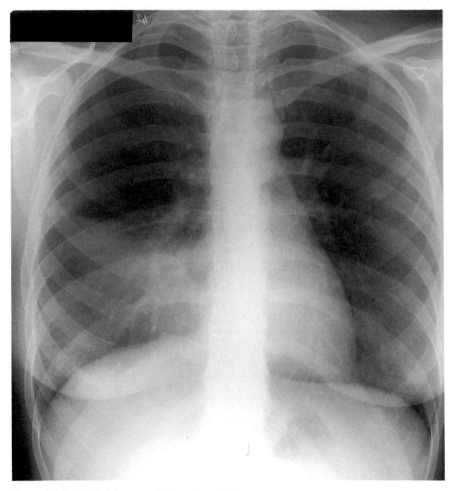

Figure 15.7. *Middle lobe consolidation. The right heart border is ill defined.*

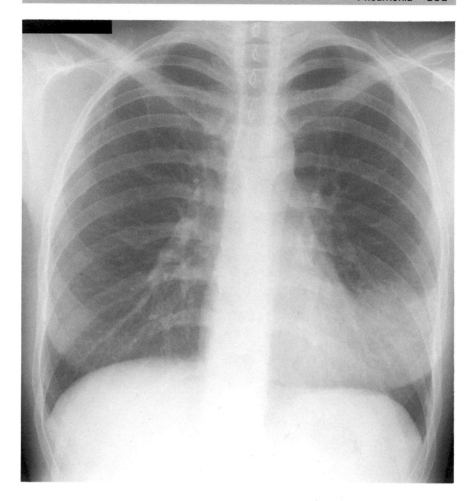

Figure 15.8. *Left upper lobe consolidation. There is increased shadowing in the lower zone of the left lung. Part of the left heart border is ill defined, indicating that the consolidation is in the lingular segment of the left upper lobe.*

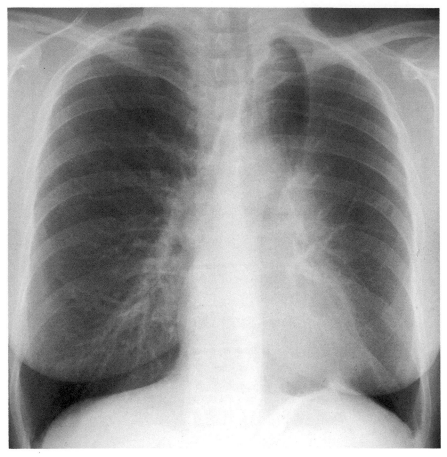

Figure 15.9. *Left upper lobe collapse and consolidation. There is diffuse shadowing in the left lung. The left heart border is ill defined indicating that the abnormality is in the upper lobe.*

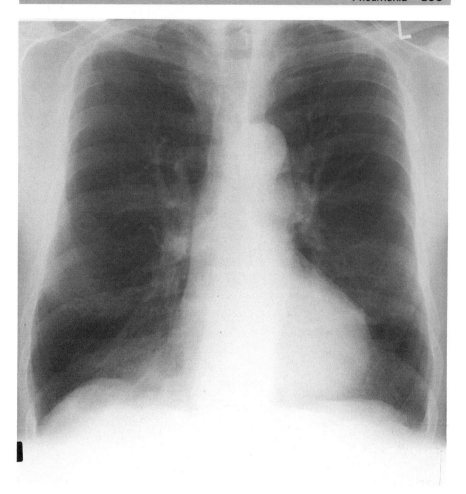

Figure 15.10. *Right lower lobe consolidation with some collapse. There is shadowing in the lower zone of the right lung and the medial part of the right hemidiaphragm is not sharply defined.*

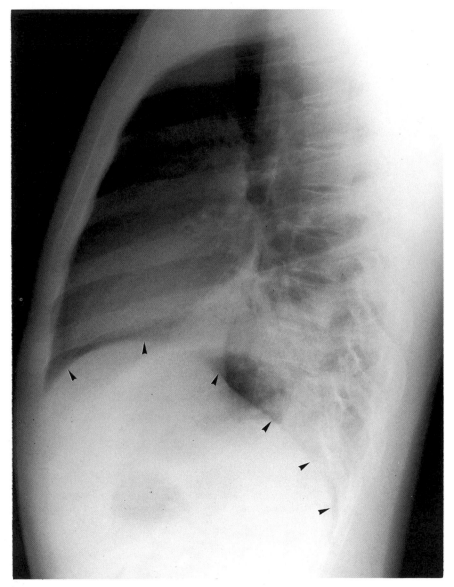

Figure 15.11. *Lateral radiograph of the same patient as in Fig 15.6. Three abnormalities on this view confirm that there is consolidation in the left lower lobe: (1) the upper surface of the right hemidiaphragm (arrowheads) is visible but that of the left hemidiaphragm is not. (2) The area behind the heart is more opaque (whiter) than the area behind the sternum, (3) the lower vertebral bodies appear more opaque than those in the upper thorax.*

KEY POINTS

- An AP radiograph may magnify the heart and suggest spurious cardiac enlargement.

- A poor inspiration may suggest spurious cardiac enlargement or spurious basal consolidation.

- A small pneumothorax is most easily seen on an expiration film.

- The demonstration of a simple rib fracture is not important. Oblique films are not indicated. A chest radiograph is obtained primarily to exclude a pleural or pulmonary complication.

- Both heart borders and both hemidiaphragms are normally clearly visible. Loss of clarity at any of these sites raises the probability of adjacent lung consolidation.

Reference

1. Armstrong P. Chest; In Keats TE (ed) *Emergency Radiology* 2nd edition. Year Book Medical Publishers, Chicago, 1989.

16 ABDOMEN

TRAUMA

Plain abdominal radiography is rarely indicated when investigating a blunt or penetrating injury. Current practice is to refer the patient directly for an ultrasound or CT examination. Many centres in Britain utilize ultrasound as the first imaging investigation with subsequent selective referral to CT. Practice does vary, and in North America for example, some departments exclude ultrasound in favour of immediate referral to CT.

A description of the possible findings on plain abdominal radiography, essentially an out of date investigation, is not useful.

ACUTE ABDOMINAL PAIN

Plain abdominal radiography continues to be useful in the investigation of patients presenting with acute abdominal pain. This chapter provides:

- Basic guidelines indicating when to request plain films
- Brief summaries of the role of diagnostic radiology in patients attending with suspected perforation, intestinal obstruction, or acute renal colic.

Guidelines for the radiological investigation of acute abdominal pain

There may be confusion as to when to request plain films.

Radiography is useful in the diagnosis of :

■ Perforation – supine abdomen and erect chest radiographs.

■ Obstruction – supine abdomen and erect chest radiographs (Refs 2 and 3). Some centres also obtain an erect abdominal film.

■ Renal colic – supine abdominal radiograph.

Ultrasound should be the first imaging procedure when the following are suspected:

■ Biliary disease.

■ Aortic aneurysm.

Plain abdominal radiography is *not* indicated for:

■ 'Non-specific' abdominal pain.

■ Gastroenteritis.

■ Constipation.

■ Acute appendicitis.

■ Urinary retention.

■ Pancreatitis.

■ Acute urinary tract infection.

■ Diarrhoea.

■ Acute peptic ulceration.

■ Haematemesis/melaena.

■ Biliary disease.

Perforation

Radiography:

■ Very small quantities (sometimes as little as 1.0 ml) of free air can be demonstrated (ref. 1).

■ The most useful radiograph is a well-penetrated erect chest film (Fig. 16.1).

■ If a patient is too unwell to sit up, then an abdominal film in the decubitus position utilizing a horizontal x-ray beam should be obtained (Fig. 16.2).

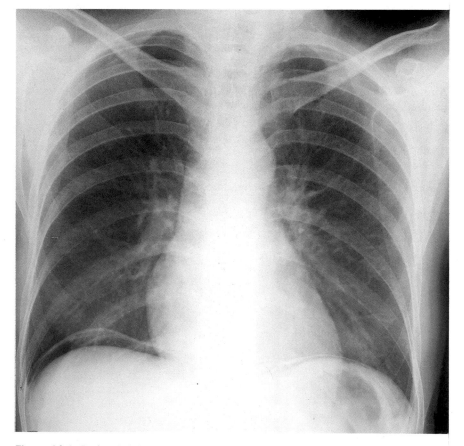

Figure 16.1. *Perforation. Air is present under both hemidiaphragms. A well penetrated erect chest film is the single most useful radiograph for the demonstration of free intraperitoneal air.*

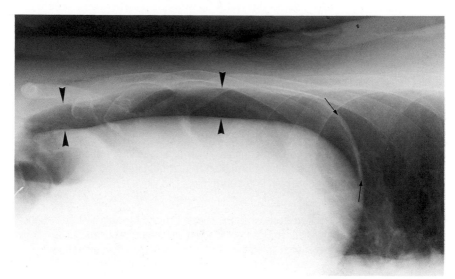

Figure 16.2. *This patient presented with abdominal pain but was too unwell to sit up. A lateral decubitus film was obtained. A large amount of free intraperitoneal air is shown (between arrowheads) above the lateral surface of the liver. The air outlines the undersurface of the right dome of the diaphragm (arrows).*

Intestinal obstruction

Radiography:

■ The most useful radiographs are an erect chest and a supine abdomen (refs 2, 3).

■ The chest film may disclose intrathoracic disease (e.g. pneumonia) which can present as acute abdominal pain (ref. 4).

■ Some centres regard an erect abdominal film as unnecessary, arguing that it rarely adds any additional useful information to that obtained from the supine view (ref. 1). Other centres obtain an erect abdominal film since it may occasionally be useful in demonstrating:

    ▨ Multiple small bowel fluid levels when the supine film shows relatively little evidence of small bowel distension. This can occur when a mechanical obstruction is present and there is a large amount of fluid within the obstructed small bowel loops.

    ▨ The 'string of beads' sign (see below).

Interpretation:

■ **Dilated small bowel with a complete absence of colon gas** suggests a complete, or nearly complete, mechanical obstruction to the small bowel (Fig. 16.3)

■ **Dilated small bowel with gas in an undistended colon** suggests either:

    ▨ A mechanical, but incomplete obstruction to the small bowel (Fig. 16.4).

    ▨ A localized adynamic ileus (Fig. 16.5).

■ **Dilated small bowel with gas in a distended colon** can indicate either:

    ▨ A mechanical obstruction to the large bowel (Fig. 16.6).

    ▨ A generalized adynamic ileus (Fig. 16.7).

■ **The 'string of beads sign'** invariably indicates a mechanical obstruction to the small bowel (ref. 5). This sign:

    ▨ Is seen on an abdominal film taken in the erect position (Fig. 16.8).

    ▨ Occurs when dilated small bowel loops are almost completely filled with fluid, and small bubbles of gas – a string of beads – are trapped in the folds along the superior wall of the distended intestine.

    ▨ Is rarely seen in a patient with an adynamic ileus because there is usually much less fluid in the small bowel.

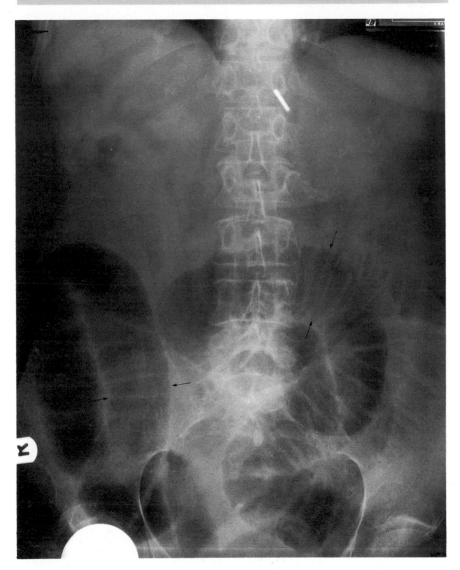

Figure 16.3. *Complete mechanical small bowel obstruction. There are dilated loops of small bowel (arrows). Some loops measure 50 mm in diameter, whereas the upper limit of normal is 30 mm. There is no gas within the large bowel.*

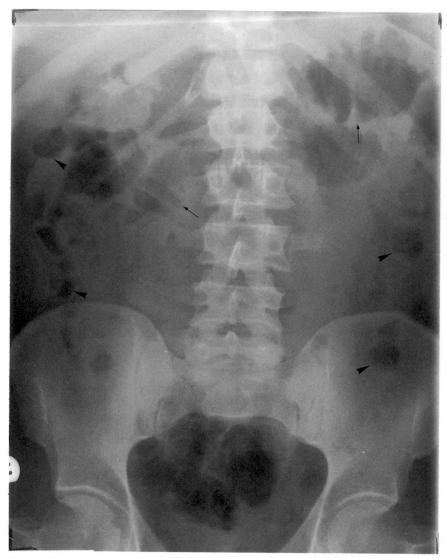

Figure 16.4. *Incomplete mechanical small bowel obstruction. There are several dilated loops of small bowel (arrows). The loop in the left upper quadrant measures 60 mm in diameter. Gas is present in the undistended large bowel (arrowheads).*

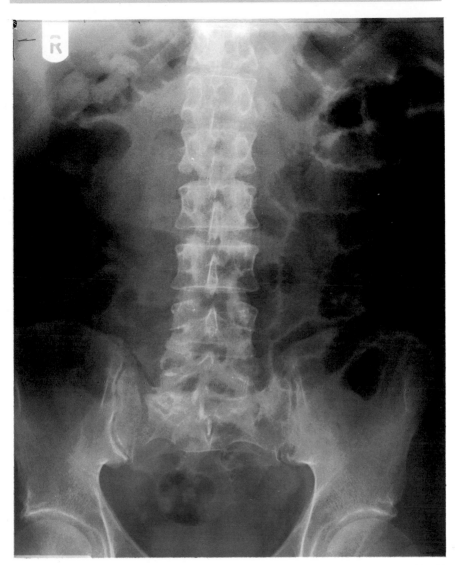

Figure 16.5. *Localized adynamic ileus. There are multiple loops of distended small bowel in the left lumbar region. This abnormal appearance was produced by acute ureteric colic.*

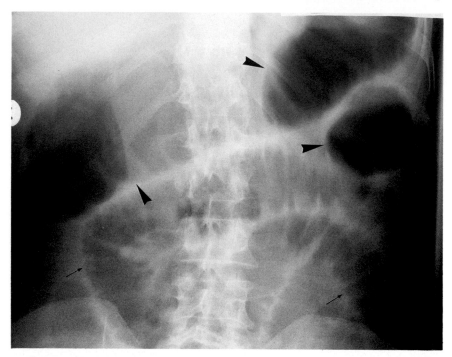

Figure 16.6. *Mechanical obstruction to the large bowel. There are dilated loops of small bowel (arrows). The transverse colon and proximal descending colon are dilated (arrowheads). There is no distension of the sigmoid colon. These findings indicate a mechanical obstruction to the left side of the large bowel.*

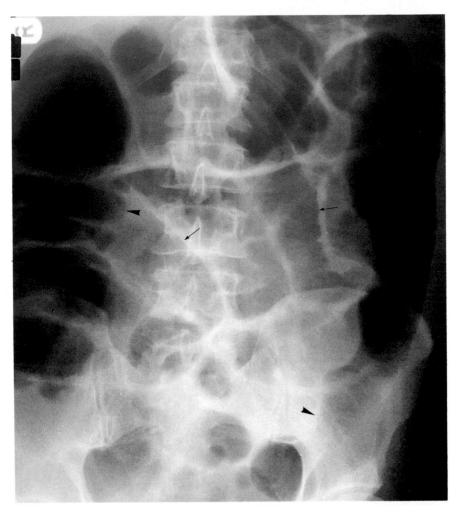

Figure 16.7. *Generalized adynamic ileus. There are dilated loops of small bowel (arrows). The entire large bowel (arrowheads) is also dilated.*

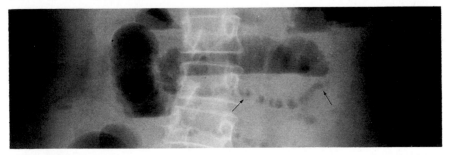

Figure 16.8. *The 'string of beads' sign. This finding (arrow) is only seen on an erect film. It is virtually pathognomonic of a mechanical obstruction to the small bowel (ref. 5).*

Renal colic

■ A plain film is helpful if there is an obvious opaque calculus in the line of the ureter, but less helpful if the film appears normal. A calculus may be hidden over bone, be confused with a pelvic phlebolith, or may not be radio-opaque. In these instances a limited intravenous urogram (IVU) – often one film only – may be necessary.

■ A limited IVU is highly accurate in confirming or excluding a calculus (Fig. 16.9).

Note: Some centres utilize the combination of a plain film and an ultrasound examination to replace the IVU. This approach might appear to be logical but:

■ Ultrasound has a false negative rate as high as 30% in acute renal colic. The error rate is highest when ultrasound is performed shortly after the onset of symptoms (ref. 6)

■ Even if the ultrasound examination is considered to be normal, then a limited IVU will still be necessary

■ For these reasons relatively few centres have adopted a protocol which uses plain films and ultrasound only.

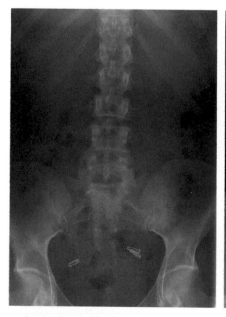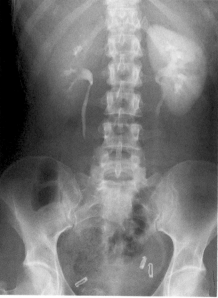

Figure 16.9. *Ureteric colic. A limited IVU (in this case only two films were necessary) confirms the clinical diagnosis. The plain film on the left does not show a definite calculus. A single film, taken 10 minutes after injection of the contrast medium, demonstrates obstruction to the left collecting system. (Sterilisation clips are projected over the pelvis.)*

KEY POINTS

Trauma

- Plain abdominal radiography not indicated.
- Ultrasound and/or CT are more useful.

Acute abdominal pain

- Perforation – 1.0 ml of free air can be demonstrated.
- Intestinal obstruction – analysis of the gas pattern in the small bowel and large intestine will indicate whether a mechanical obstruction or a paralytic ileus is present.
- Renal colic – a limited IVU (usually only two films) is highly accurate in confirming or excluding the diagnosis.

References

1. Miller RE, Nelson SW. The roentgenologic demonstration of tiny amounts of free intraperitoneal gas: experimental and clinical studies. *Am J Roent* 1971, **112:** 574–585.
2. Field S, Guy P, Upsdell SM, Scourfield AE. The erect abdominal radiograph in the acute abdomen: should its routine use be abandoned? *Br Med J* 1985, **290:** 1934–1936.
3. Jelinek GA and Banham NDG. Reducing the use of plain abdominal radiographs in an Emergency Department. *Arch Emerg Med* 1990, **7:** 241–245.
4. Hayward MW, Hayward C, Ennis WP, Roberts CJ. A pilot evaluation of radiography of the acute abdomen. *Clin Radiol* 1984, **35:** 289–291.
5. Gammill SL, Nice CM. Air fluid levels: their occurrence in normal patients and their role in the analysis of ileus. *Surgery* 1972, **71:** 771–780.
6. Platt JF, Rubin JM, Ellis JH. Acute renal obstruction: evaluation with intrarenal duplex Doppler and conventional ultrasound. *Radiology* 1993, **186:** 685–688.

17 PENETRATING FOREIGN BODIES

GLASS

Detection

■ **All glass is radio opaque.** The visibility of glass (Fig. 17.1) is **not** dependent on its lead content (refs 1, 2)

■ Radiographic technique is important. A soft tissue exposure is essential when glass fragments are being sought.

■ The area of interest needs to be projected away from overlying bone by using two or more projections (Figs 17.2 and 17.3).

■ It is often necessary to use a magnifying glass, otherwise very small fragments will be overlooked.

Pitfall: A patient falls from a height through a glass roof and sustains a laceration to the upper thigh. The force of the fall may drive a glass fragment deep into the muscle well away from the skin laceration. With this history it would be insufficient to obtain films solely of the area immediately adjacent to the wound. Whenever there is a history of a considerable force then the radiographs must be checked to see that they include the deep tissues.

Removal

Plain radiography is excellent at detecting all metal and glass foreign bodies(FBs). On the other hand it may be of limited assistance when the surgeon attempts to remove a fragment situated deep in the tissues.

Ultrasound can be very helpful in assisting with the removal of any radio-opaque FB (ref. 3)

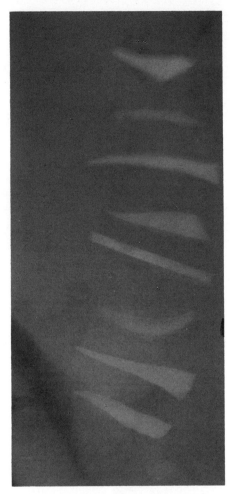

Figure 17.1. Radiograph of different types of glass placed in a piece of meat. All types of glass will be shown on plain films, but some types (e.g. light-bulb) are less radio-opaque than others. From above downwards: windscreen, light bulb, soft drinks bottle, milk bottle, wine bottle, wine glass, beer bottle, beer glass. (From ref. 2, with permission.)

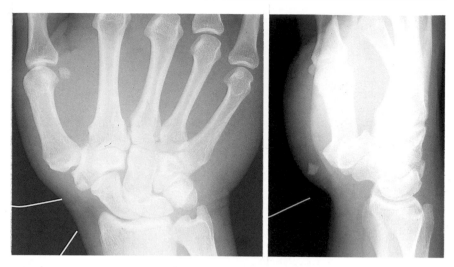

Figure 17.2. *A dense glass fragment is hidden by bone on the PA radiograph. When it is projected clear of bone it is easy to see.*

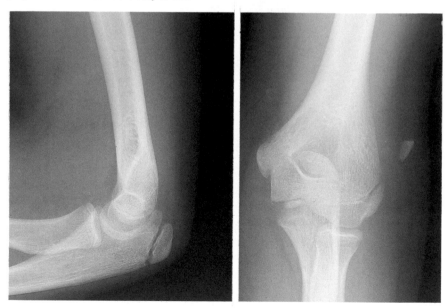

Figure 17.3. *Two views are always necessary. The glass fragment is not seen on the lateral view. It is hidden by the overlying bone.*

WOOD OR PLASTIC

Detection

- Wood splinters are sometimes radio-opaque (ref. 4) but can be very difficult to detect with plain film radiography. Occasionally a splinter will be seen on an x-ray film if the fragment has paint on its surface (Fig. 17.4).

- Detection of wood splinters, thorns and plastic is best carried out using ultrasound (refs 3, 5 and 6).

Removal

Plain film radiography is not useful for removal of wood or plastic. Ultrasound can be very helpful (ref. 3). CT or MRI are also available in exceptionally difficult cases.

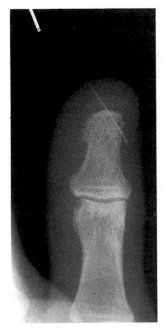

Figure 17.4. *This splinter of wood is seen because it had a thick coat of paint on its surface. It is usually very difficult to visualize wooden splinters and thorns on a radiograph.*

FOREIGN BODIES IN THE ORBIT

Detection

■ Most FBs are diagnosed with slit lamp ophthalmoscopy. Detection does not depend solely on an imaging investigation. When necessary plain radiography, ultrasound or CT can be of assistance.

■ **Metal or glass fragments:**

  ▪ Plain radiography.

  ▪ The standard views: two frontal projections, with upward and downward gaze, and a lateral.

  ▪ The movement of a FB on upward and downward gaze will indicate whether and where it is situated within the globe (Fig. 17.5).

■ **Wood or plastic fragments**

  ▪ Ultrasound is useful. The accuracy of detection is in large part dependent on an experienced operator and the quality of the equipment (ref. 7).

  ▪ CT is an alternative to ultrasound (Fig. 17.6). CT is sensitive, shows the retrobulbar space better than ultrasound, and is less operator-dependent (ref. 7).

Removal

Either ultrasound or CT can assist with accurate localization (refs 7 and 8).

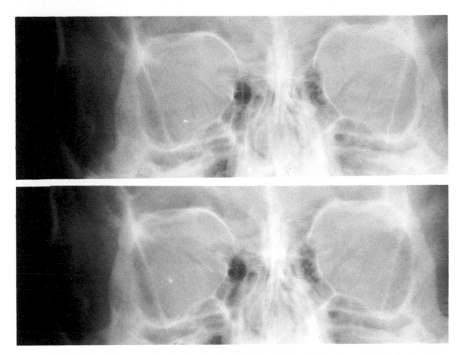

Figure 17.5. *There is a metallic foreign body within the right orbit. Radiograph obtained with the patient looking down (top) and looking up (bottom). The position of the fragment changes. This confirms that it lies within the globe.*

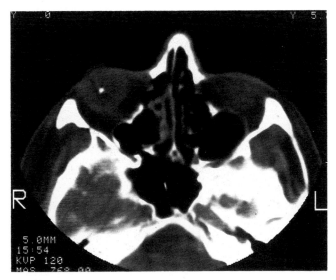

Figure 17.6. *CT scan demonstrating the precise position of a metallic foreign body within the right eye.*

KEY POINTS

Foreign bodies in soft tissue

■ **Detection:**

  ▩ For radio-opaque FBs use plain films.

  ▩ For non radio-opaque FBs use ultrasound.

■ **Removal –precise localization:**

  ▩ For all FBs use ultrasound, or CT or MRI in a few exceptionally difficult cases.

Foreign bodies in the orbit

■ Clinical examination with slit lamp ophthalmoscopy will detect the majority of FBs.

■ Imaging is *secondary* to ophthalmoscopy.

■ Imaging.

  ▩ Metal fragments – plain radiography.

  ▩ Wood or plastic – US or CT.

References

1. Tandberg D. Glass in the hand and foot. Will an x-ray show it? *J Am Med Assoc* 1982, **248:** 1872–1874.
2. de Lacey G, Evans R, Sandin B. Penetrating injuries: how easy is it to see glass (and plastic) on radiographs? *Br J Radiol* 1985, **58:** 27–30.
3. Gilbert FJ, Campbell RSD, Bayliss AP.The role of ultrasound in the detection of non-radiopaque foreign bodies. *Clin Radiol* 1990, **41:** 109–112.
4. Roobottom CA, Weston MJ. The detection of foreign bodies in soft tissue – comparison of conventional and digital radiography. *Clin Radiol* 1994, **49**: 330–332.
5. Ginsburg MJ, Ellis GL, Flom LL. Detection of soft-tissue foreign bodies by plain radiography, xerography, computed tomography, and ultrasonography. *Ann Emerg Med* 1990, **19:** 701–703.
6. Schlesinger AE, Hernandez RJ. Diseases of the musculoskeletal system in children: imaging with CT, sonography, and MR. *Am J Radiol* 1992, **158:** 729–741.
7. McElvanney AM, Fielder AR. Intraocular foreign body missed by radiography. *Br Med J* 1993, **306:** 1060–1061.
8. Etherington R.J., Hourihan M.D. Localisation of intraocular and intraorbital foreign bodies using computed tomography. *Clin Radiol* 1989, **40:** 610–614.

18 SWALLOWED FOREIGN BODIES

SHARP OR POTENTIALLY POISONOUS OBJECTS

■ Sharp objects need to be confirmed or excluded by radiography (Fig. 18.1).

■ Very occasionally the contents of a swallowed disc battery may leak out. Most modern disc batteries contain sodium or potassium hydroxide which is corrosive. Some contain mercury which is poisonous (refs 1 and 2).

Radiography

■ An abdominal radiograph (Fig 18.2).

■ If the foreign body (FB) is not seen, then frontal and lateral chest radiographs (to include the neck) are obtained.

■ If a swallowed battery is demonstrated on the abdominal film then this radiograph should be repeated every 24 hours. If there is any sign of delay, or disintegration, then endoscopic or surgical removal needs urgent consideration.

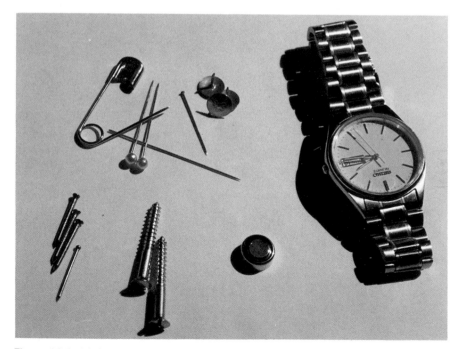

Figure 18.1. *It is important that sharp or poisonous objects are identified. If there is an appropriate history then abdominal radiography is indicated.*

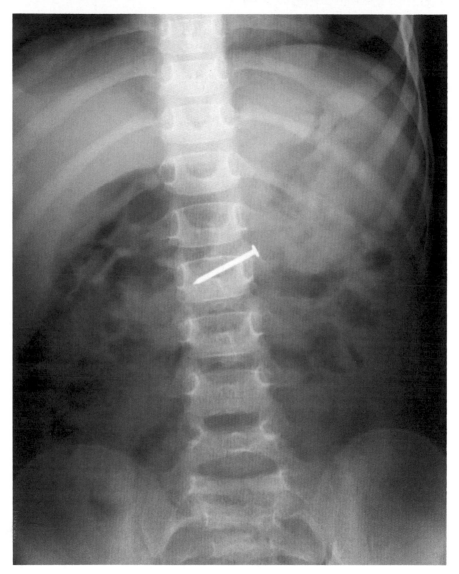

Figure 18.2. *Swallowed nail. This was passed uneventfully.*

COINS AND SMALL BLUNT OBJECTS

Children

■ There is no danger to the child if the coin lies within the stomach or the intestine.

■ A radiograph of the abdomen (Fig. 18.3) is clinically unnecessary and represents unjustified radiation exposure (refs 1, 3).

■ Occasionally a coin may lodge in the oesophagus (Fig. 18.4). Some of these patients may remain asymptomatic. There is danger of erosion of the mucosa by the coin (ref. 2).

Radiography:

■ A single AP radiograph of the chest to include the neck.

■ **No abdominal radiography** (refs 2, 4 and 5).

■ If the chest/neck film is normal then the parents can be reassured that the coin has passed into the gut, it will cause no harm, and will be excreted within the next few days.

Adults

■ In the adult, the vertebral bodies and mediastinal structures are dense and superimposed over the oesophagus on the AP view. A single AP radiograph of the chest and neck may not show a metallic density (Fig. 18.5).

■ On the lateral view the mid and lower oesophagus are not obscured by dense tissues. A radio-opaque FB will be obvious (Fig. 18.6).

Radiography:

■ Well-penetrated AP and lateral chest films, to include the neck.

■ **No need for abdominal radiography.**

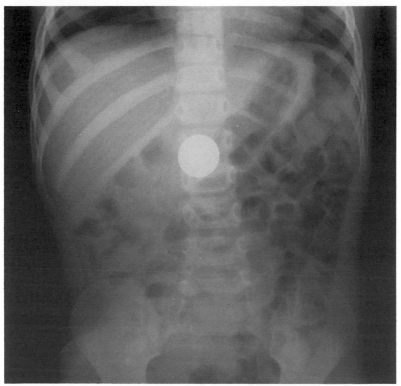

Figure 18.3. *Swallowed coin. Abdominal radiography is not indicated. It represents unjustified radiation exposure. A coin that has passed out of the gullet will do no harm.*

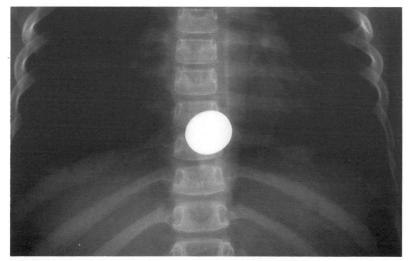

Figure 18.4. *Swallowed coin. Chest radiography is indicated. The coin is impacted at the lower end of the oesophagus. Very occasionally it will remain impacted and erode the mucosa.*

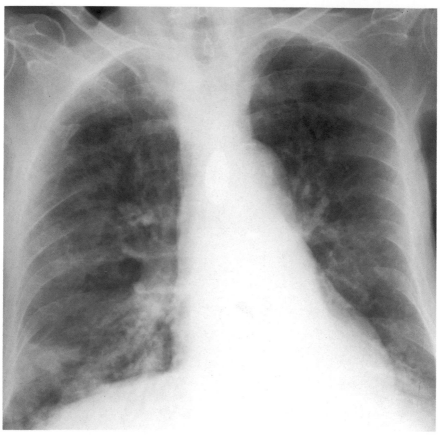

Figure 18.5. *Adult. A swallowed coin has impacted at the level of the aortic arch. It is only just visible on this AP radiograph.*

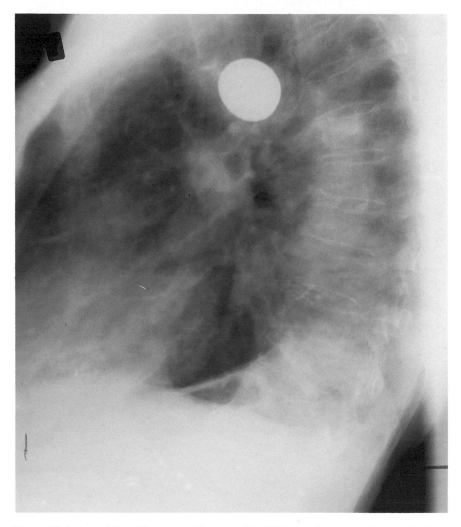

Figure 18.6. *Lateral film of the same patient as in Fig. 18.5.* **A radio-opaque foreign body which impacts in the adult oesophagus is most easily seen on the lateral view.**

LARGE OBJECTS

■ A large object (such as a dental appliance) may lodge in the cervical or thoracic oesophagus (Figs 18.7 and 18.8). If it remains impacted it may erode the mucosa (ref. 6).

■ **Not all dentures are radio-opaque**, and plain films may therefore appear normal.

Radiography

■ Well-penetrated AP and lateral chest films, to include the neck.

■ If these films are normal then an abdominal radiograph should be obtained.

■ If this film is normal, and the clinical history remains suggestive, then a barium swallow or endoscopy will be necessary.

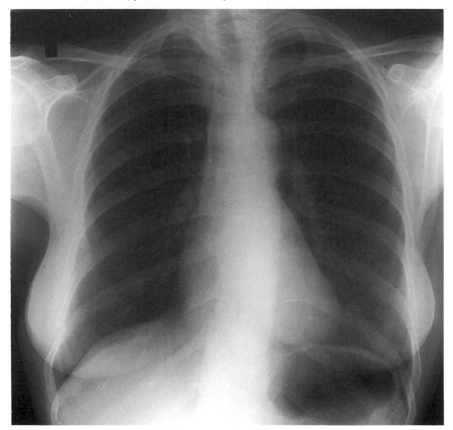

Figure 18.7. *This patient claimed to have swallowed her dentures. No evidence of a foreign body on the PA chest radiograph. She was discharged.*

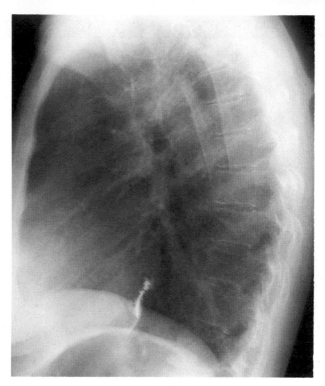

Figure 18.8. *Same patient as in Fig 18.7. The patient was recalled for a lateral film. The impacted dentures are now obvious.*

FISH AND CHICKEN BONES

■ Penetrating bones tend to lodge in the laryngeal pharynx or upper oesophagus (refs 6, 7).

■ It can be helpful to know the exact type of fish that was eaten, as not all fish bones are calcified, and the radio-opacity of the bones will vary (ref. 8):

    ■ **Readily visible** – Cod, Haddock, Cole fish, Lemon Sole, Gurnard.

    ■ **More difficult to see** – Grey Mullet, Plaice, Monkfish, Red snapper.

    ■ **Not visible** – Herring, (kipper), Salmon, Mackerel, Trout, Pike.

Radiography

■ A soft tissue lateral radiograph of the neck (refs 1, 7).

■ Direct signs (a bone) or indirect signs (swelling or gas due to a perforation) may be identified (Fig. 18.9). Occasionally, the films may be difficult to interpret: a bone may be mistaken for a calcified laryngeal cartilage, and vice versa (Fig. 18.10).

■ It is important to maintain a low threshold for proceeding to endoscopy.

■ Any patient considered well enough to be sent home following seemingly normal plain films should be told to re-attend the next day if symptoms persist. Patients who re-attend should be seen there and then by an ear, nose and throat specialist.

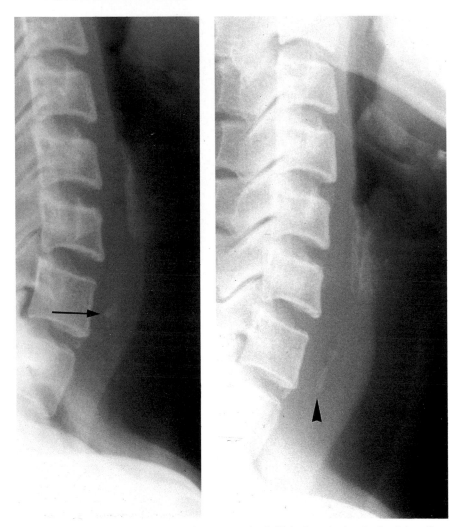

Figure 18.9. *Impacted chicken bone. On presentation (left) the bone lay in a horizontal position (arrow) and was not recognized. Several days later (right) the bone is easy to identify as it now lies vertically (arrowhead). Note the soft tissue swelling and faint bubbles of gas, indicating an abscess around a perforation. (Acknowledgement – The authors thank the editor of* Imaging *for giving permission to reproduce this figure from: Remedios D, Charlesworth C and de Lacey G,* Imaging *1993,* **5:** *171–179.)*

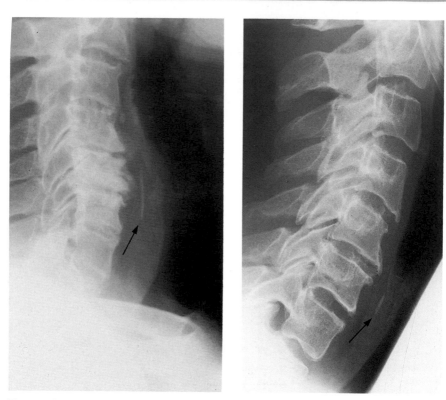

Figure 18.10. Pitfalls: *the patient on the left has swallowed a chicken bone (arrow). The patient on the right shows a somewhat similar appearance (arrow), but this is due to ossification in the cricoid cartilage. When in doubt an experienced observer should be consulted.*

KEY POINTS

■ **Sharp or poisonous objects:**

  ▨ Abdominal radiograph. If this is normal, obtain well-penetrated AP and lateral chest films.

■ **Coins**

  ▨ Abdominal radiography is *not* indicated.

  ▨ Children – a single well-penetrated AP chest radiograph to include neck.

  ▨ Adults – well-penetrated AP and lateral chest radiographs to include neck.

■ **Large objects**

  ▨ Frontal and lateral chest films. If normal obtain an abdominal radiograph.

  ▨ If this is also normal, then consider a barium swallow or endoscopy.

■ **Fish and Chicken bones**

  ▨ A lateral neck radiograph is indicated.

  ▨ If the radiograph is normal and the patient is fit for discharge, then clear instructions need to be given. For example:

    'If symptoms are still present after 24 hours then please return for an examination by the ear, nose and throat specialist'.

  ▨ There should be a low threshold for proceeding to endoscopy.

References

1. Remedios D, Charlesworth C, deLacey G. Imaging of foreign bodies. *Imaging* 1993, **5:** 171–179.
2. Cooke MW, Glucksman EE. Swallowed coins. *Br Med J* 1991, **302:** 1607.
3. Park C. Seeing is believing. *Br Med J* 1993, **307:** 1010.
4. Stringer MD, Capps SNJ. Rationalising the management of swallowed coins in children. *Br Med J* 1991, **302:** 1321–1322.
5. Swallowed coins. Editorial. *Lancet* 1989, **2:** 659–660.
6. Remsen K, Biller HF, Lawson W, Som, L. Unusual presentations of penetrating foreign bodies of the upper aerodigestive tract. *Ann Otol Rhinol Laryngol (Suppl)* 1983 July–August, **105:** 32–44.
7. Herdman RCD, Saeed SR, Hinton EA. The lateral soft tissue x-ray in accident and emergency medicine. *Arch Emerg Med* 1991, **8:** 149–156.
8. Ell SR, Sprigg A. The radio-opacity of fishbones – species variation. *Clin Radiol* 1991, **44:** 104–107.

19 PARTICULAR PAEDIATRIC POINTS

Several aspects of paediatric radiology are referred to and illustrated elsewhere:

- The shoulder in Chapter 4, page 54;
- The elbow in Chapter 5, page 78;
- The pelvis in Chapter 10, page 134;
- The foot in Chapter 13, page 169;
- Swallowed foreign bodies in Chapter 18, page 218.

GREENSTICK, TORUS AND PLASTIC BOWING FRACTURES

These fractures differ in appearance from fractures in adults mainly because the child's skeleton is elastic. In addition the periosteum is not only elastic but it is also very thick.

Greenstick fracture

Results from an angulation force. There is a break in one cortex of the bone. The opposite cortex remains intact (Figs 19.1 and 19.2). There is usually some degree of angulation at the fracture site, though this can be subtle. These injuries are rarely overlooked.

Torus fracture

Results from a longitudinal compression force and is a variation of a greenstick fracture. There are microfractures of the trabeculae at the injured site. Instead of a break in the cortex there is just slight buckling (Figs 19.2 and 19.3). There is little or no angulation. The commonest sites for this injury are the distal radius and ulna, usually following a fall on the outstretched hand. These injuries are often subtle.

Plastic bowing fracture

In addition to the above injuries a bone may simply bend with no obvious break in the cortex. These plastic bowing fractures usually involve the radius or ulna (Fig. 19.4). They can be extremely difficult to diagnose as differences in radiographic positioning can mimic a slightly bent bone. Sometimes these fractures are only recognized when the child re-attends, and repeat films show healing periosteal new bone along the shaft.

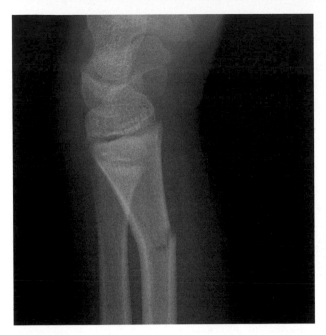

Figure 19.1. *Greenstick fracture of the radius. There is slight angulation.*

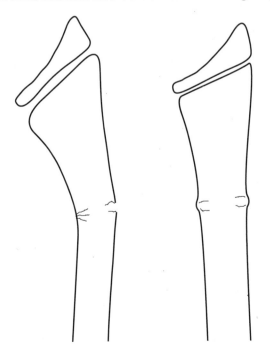

Figure 19.2. *Greenstick fracture – cortical break with angulation (left). Torus fracture – cortical buckling but no angulation (right).*

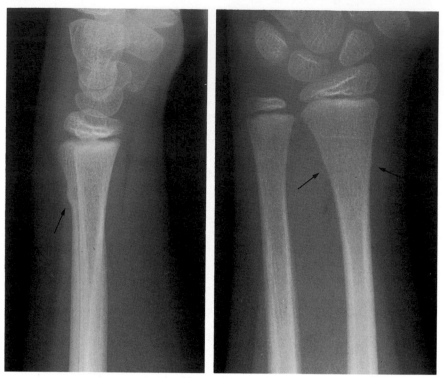

Figure 19.3. *Torus fracture. Buckling of the radial cortex is best seen on the lateral view. There is no angulation.*

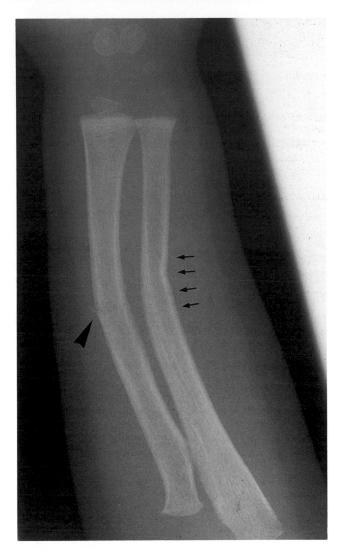

Figure 19.4. *Plastic bowing fracture. The ulna appears bent (arrows). There is also a greenstick fracture of the radius (arrowhead).*

GROWTH PLATE INJURIES: SALTER–HARRIS FRACTURES

These fractures involve the growth plate of the unfused skeleton.

The Salter–Harris classification (Fig. 19.5) is based on the clinical importance of the injury. A Salter–Harris type 1 injury has a good prognosis whereas type 5 has a poor prognosis. Failure to recognise that the epiphyseal plate is involved by a fracture may result in suboptimal treatment. There is a risk of premature fusion of the growth plate resulting in limb shortening. If only part of the plate is injured, unequal growth might also lead to deformity and disability.

Type 1 is a fracture across the growth plate (Fig 19.6). Sometimes there is only very slight displacement of the epiphysis from the metaphysis, in which case it is impossible to detect the injury on the radiograph. Prognosis is very good.

Types 2–4 represent various patterns of fracture involving the growth plate and the adjacent metaphysis and/or epiphysis (Figs 19.7–19.9). Type 4 may be associated with premature fusion of part of the growth plate.

Type 5 is an impaction fracture of the entire growth plate. There is little or no malalignment. For this reason it can be extremely difficult to diagnose from the radiographs. This is the most significant of all the Salter–Harris injuries since the plate may fuse prematurely with consequent limb shortening. Diagnosis and subsequent management depends on a high degree of suspicion following clinical examination.

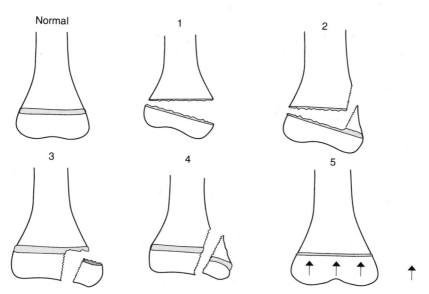

Figure 19.5. *Epiphyseal fractures. The Salter–Harris classification.*

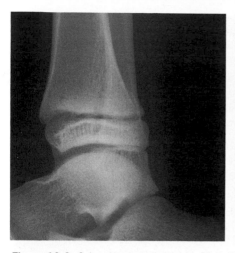

Figure 19.6. *Salter–Harris type 1 injury. There is widening of the tibial epiphyseal plate anteriorly and laterally. The epiphysis is not displaced.*

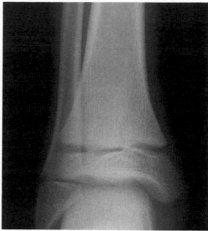

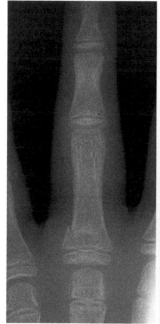

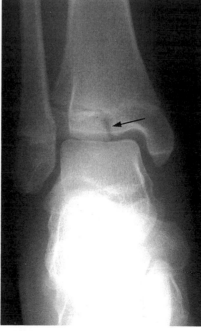

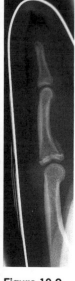

Figure 19.7. *Salter–Harris type 2 injury. There is a fracture through the metaphysis of the proximal phalanx extending into the epiphyseal plate.*

Figure 19.8. *Salter–Harris type 3 injury. There is a fracture through the distal tibial epiphysis extending into the epiphyseal plate. The lateral aspect of the growth plate is widened.*

Figure 19.9. *Salter–Harris type 4 injury. The fracture involves the epiphyseal plate, the epiphysis and the metaphysis.*

PULLED ELBOW

Also known as Nursemaid's elbow.

■ A sudden pull on the hand with the elbow extended may cause the radial head to sublux through the annular ligament. The clinical diagnosis is usually obvious, and reduction is achieved simply by supinating the forearm. A successful reduction is accompanied by immediate relief of symptoms.

■ When the clinical features are typical, radiography is not indicated. Furthermore, radiography will not be helpful as a large gap between the bony ends of the radial and humeral metaphyses is normal, due to the unossified radial head and capitellum.

TODDLER'S FRACTURE

This injury results when a toddler begins to walk and falls with one leg stationary whilst the other leg twists. Twisting results in a spiral fracture of the tibia (Fig. 19.10). Displacement of the fragments may be minimal and the fracture difficult to detect.

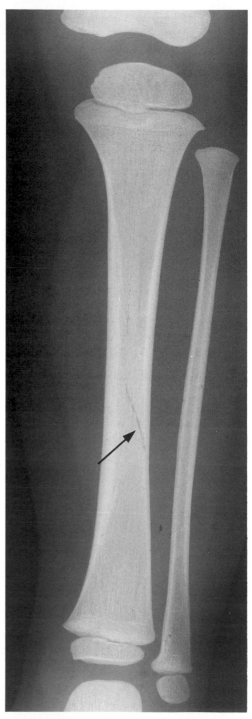

Figure 19.10. *Toddler's fracture. Spiral fracture of the middle third of the tibia.*

THE PAEDIATRIC SKULL

There are numerous normal appearances which may be confusing. It is often necessary to consult *Keats' Atlas* (ref. 1) or to seek the opinion of an experienced observer. Even then there will be occasions when it will still be difficult to distinguish between a normal finding and a fracture.

Additional sutures

A child's skull may show one or more additional sutures, which rarely persist into adult life.

Some common accessory sutures and synchondroses:

■ Metopic – between the two halves of the frontal bone (Fig. 19.11).

■ Spheno-occipital synchondrosis – between the posterior aspect of the sphenoid and the anterior margin of the occiput (Fig. 19.12).

■ Intraparietal – through the parietal bone (Fig. 19.13). It can be unilateral or bilateral

Widening of sutures

Following a head injury a suture may be diastased (widened) due to either a sutural fracture or intracranial haemorrhage. Sutural widening may be the only evidence of injury (Fig. 19.14).

Pitfall: The width of the normal sutures is very variable, and it is important to adopt a cautious approach when widening is observed. An experienced observer will often be able to provide reassurance that the appearance is within the normal range.

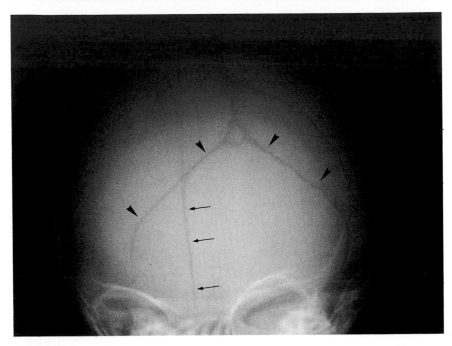

Figure 19.11. *The metopic suture (arrows) which separates the two frontal bones on this slightly rotated radiograph. The arrowheads indicate the lambdoid sutures.*

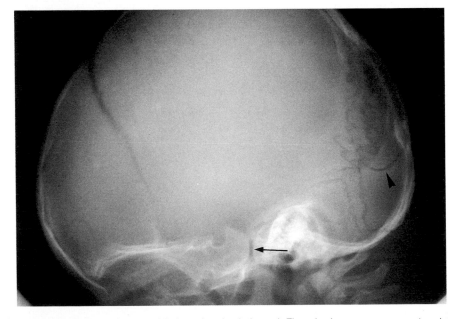

Figure 19.12. *The spheno-occipital synchondrosis (arrow). There is also an accessory suture in the occipital bone (arrowhead).*

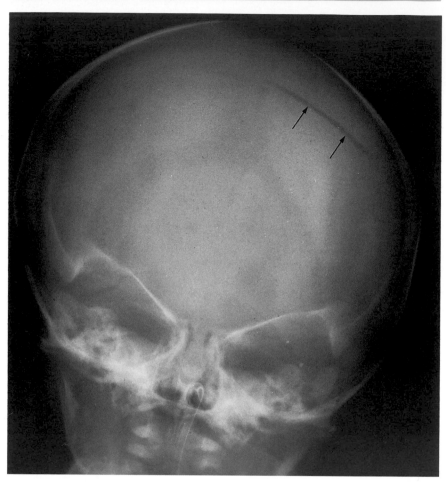

Figure 19.13. *An intraparietal suture.*

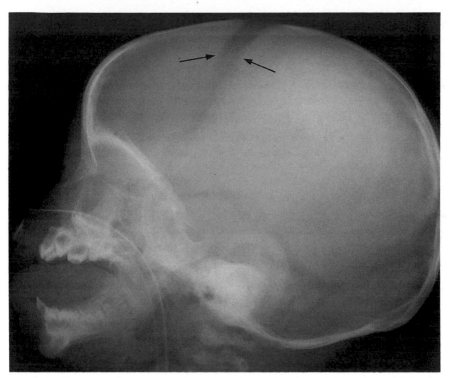

Figure 19.14. *Widening (diastasis) of the sutures due to raised intracranial pressure. This child had been violently shaken, but there had been no direct trauma to the head. A subsequent CT scan revealed extensive intracranial haemorrhage.*

PAINFUL HIP IN THE ABSENCE OF TRAUMA

Differential diagnosis

■ Children complaining of hip pain are the commonest cause of paediatric orthopaedic admissions in the UK.

■ Infants and toddlers may be brought to the Accident Department because they appear reluctant to move a leg, but without any direct hip signs or symptoms. Most of these children are eventually diagnosed as having a transient synovitis (irritable hip) which is a self-limiting condition associated with a joint effusion and presumed to be of viral aetiology. Rarely a more serious abnormality is found. This may be a septic arthritis, Perthes' disease or a slipped femoral capital epiphysis.

■ The patient's age will give some idea as to the most likely cause of hip pain, though there is overlap within the various age groups:

   ▩ **Irritable hips** occur in both sexes, throughout childhood.

   ▩ **Perthes' disease** is more common in boys. It is rare over the age of 7 years.

   ▩ **Slipped epiphysis** (SFCE) is more common in boys. It is rare under the age of 8 years.

■ It is common practice to admit most children with suspected hip pain because of the concern that a septic arthritis may be overlooked. Though septic arthritis is rare it is very important since the infection can destroy an immature femoral head within a few days. Unfortunately there are no simple clinical or blood tests that will guarantee to exclude a septic arthritis; temperature, white cell count and ESR are normal in one third of affected patients. The only certain way to exclude this condition is to obtain synovial fluid for gram stain and culture.

The investigation of the painful hip

Practice does vary between centres. However, the following is a protocol which has recently been utilised in children presenting with hip pain or a reluctance to move a leg (ref. 2).

- The patient is placed under the care of the specialist paediatric or orthopaedic team.

- On admission to the Accident Department some local anaesthetic cream is placed on the hip skin crease.

- A plain radiograph is obtained:

  - Obvious Perthes' disease or SCFE – **stop.**

  - The film appears normal – **proceed to:**

    - ❏ Immediate hip ultrasound for confirmation or exclusion of a joint effusion.

    - ❏ In every case of effusion the joint fluid is aspirated under ultrasound control. Immediate gram stains are performed. If positive start therapy. If negative the child may be safely discharged home whilst awaiting the result of culture – *provided that the family is within easy reach by telephone.*

- All children are reviewed one week later in the paediatric or orthopaedic clinic. If the pain still persists then an isotope bone scan is obtained in order to exclude early Perthes' disease or other extremely rare causes of hip pain such as pubic osteomyelitis or a bone tumour.

- Using this protocol (ref. 2) the irritable hip is transformed from the most common cause of paediatric orthopaedic hospital admission into a condition which may safely be managed as an out-patient.

INHALED FOREIGN BODY

The most commonly inhaled foreign body is food, frequently a peanut (ref. 3). A history of choking is usually obtained. Common clinical signs include cough, stridor, wheezing and sternal retraction.

- **Radiography.** PA and lateral chest films:
  - if the child is able to cooperate then the PA view should be obtained following a rapid forced expiration. Air trapping on the affected side is then more obvious (Figs 19.15 and 19.16).

- **Possible findings:**
  - area of collapse/consolidation
  - unilateral hypertransradiant lung. Due to air trapping, the affected lung appears blacker and larger than the opposite normal side (Figs 19.15 and 19.16)
  - the foreign body. This will be infrequent because peanuts and other food are not radio-opaque
  - normal appearances (ref. 4).

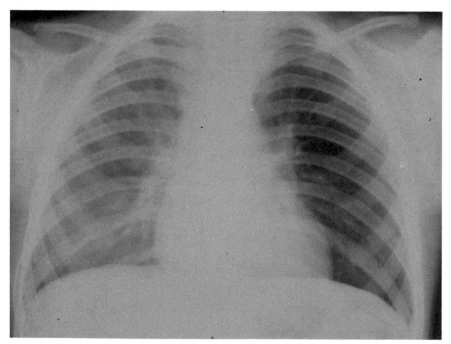

Figure 19.15. *Inhaled foreign body. Inspiration film. The left lung is hypertransradiant (i.e. blacker) when compared with the right.*

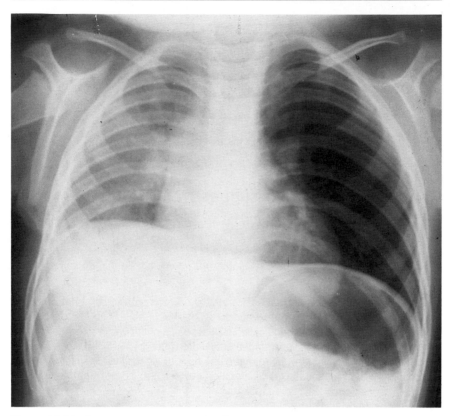

Figure 19.16. *Same patient as in Fig. 19.15. Radiograph following rapid forced expiration. The abnormal air trapping in the left lung is more obvious. (Radiographs courtesy of Dr CD Flower, Addenbrooke's Hospital, Cambridge.)*

NON-ACCIDENTAL INJURY (NAI)

■ The possibility of NAI needs to be considered in all children presenting to the Accident Department with an injury. No socio-economic group or race is exempt:

▨ 50% of cases of NAI occur before the age of 1 year.

▨ 80% occur before the age of 2 years.

■ Normal radiographs do not exclude the diagnosis. In approximately 50% of proven cases the radiographs will be normal.

Radiographic features suggestive of NAI

■ More than one fracture (Fig. 19.17). This is particularly suspicious if the stages of evolution of the fractures appear to be different, since this indicates that the injuries have occurred at different times. For example, one fracture may show a slight periosteal reaction whereas another may demonstrate mature callus formation.

■ Subperiosteal new bone formation. Periosteal reactions may result from subperiosteal bleeding caused by punching, shaking or squeezing (Fig. 19.18). Though periosteal reaction and callus formation can occur within a few days of trauma, neither will be present on the actual day of the injury. If new bone is present then it can be concluded that some days or weeks have elapsed between the injury occurring and the child being brought to the Accident Department.

Radiographic features virtually pathognomic of NAI

■ A small fracture (Fig. 19.19) at the corner of a metaphysis of a long bone. This is known as a corner (or bucket handle) fracture.

■ Rib fractures involving the posterior aspects close to the spine (Figs 19.17 and 19.18). They occur when a child is held by the chest and shaken or squeezed.

▨ Rib fractures in children under the age of 2 years are usually due to NAI.

▨ Rib fractures often result from very violent shaking episodes, and these have a recognized association with diffuse or local brain injury. The presence of rib fractures is a legitimate indication for a CT scan of the brain (Fig. 19.14), even in a child who appears neurologically normal.

■ Fractures of the pelvis, sternum, and the vertebral transverse processes. These injuries are rarely caused by an accidental injury.

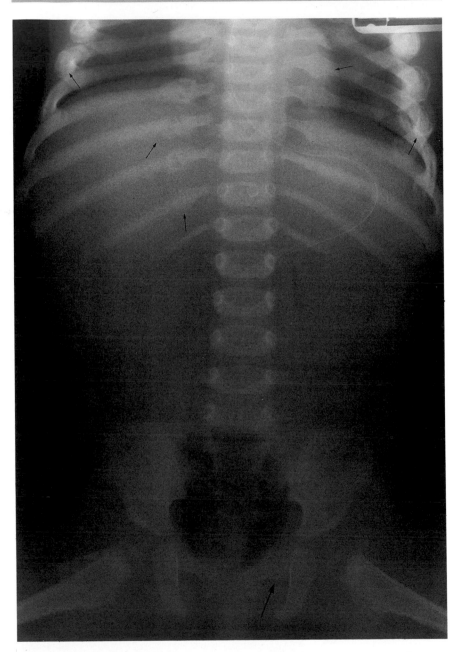

Figure 19.17. *NAI. Multiple fractures.*

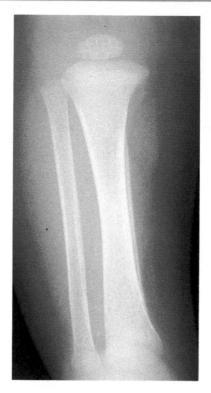

Figure 19.18. *NAI. Periosteal reactions along the medial aspect of the tibia. The child had been gripped very hard by both legs and shaken violently.*

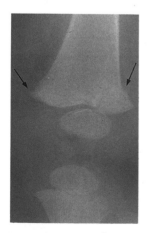

Figure 19.19. *NAI. Fractures of the distal tibial metaphysis. These represent corner (bucket handle) fractures.*

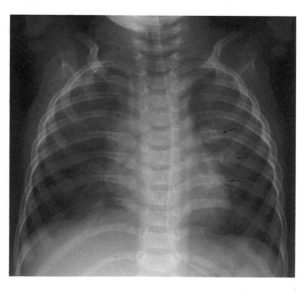

Figure 19.20. *NAI. Multiple fractures of the ribs posteriorly.*

References

1. Keats TE. *Atlas of Normal Roentgen Variants That May Simulate Disease*, 5th edn. Year Book Medical Publishers, Chicago, 1991.
2. Fink M, Berman L, Edwards D, Jacobson K. Irritable hips – is there a need for hospital admission? *Br J Radiol* 1993, **66:** 629.
3. Rothman BF, Boeckman CR. Foreign bodies in the larynx and tracheo-bronchial tree in children. *Ann Otol* 1980, **89:** 434–436.
4. Svedstrom E, Puhakka H, Kero P. How accurate is chest radiography in the diagnosis of tracheobronchial foreign bodies in children? *Pediatr Radiol* 1989, **19:** 520–522.

INDEX